Inside Alzheimer's

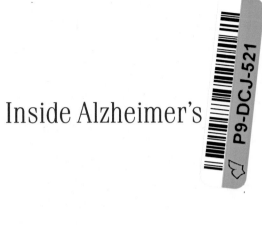

Inside Alzheimer's

How to Hear and Honor Connections with a Person who has Dementia

Nancy D. Pearce

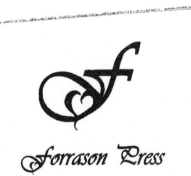

Forrason Press

Taylors, SC

First Forrason Press edition: August 2007
Second Printing: December 2007
Visit our Web site: http://www.forrasonpress.com

Library of Congress Control Number: 2006909855

ISBN-13: 978-0-9788299-0-2
ISBN-10: 0-9788299-0-5

Quantity discounts are available on bulk purchases of this book for ed-
ucational, business, or sales promotional use.
For information, please write to Customer Service, Forrason Press,
Post Office Box 1032, Taylors, SC 29687 or send your email request to
custserv@forrasonpress.com

Edited by Judith Blahnik and Sharon Creal
Cover design and typesetting by John Cole, Graphic Designer,
    Santa Fe, NM. www.johncolegrf.com
Author photo by Pat Rawlins (copyright © 2006); 864-232-2944
Manufactured in the United States of America by Vaughan Printing,
    Inc., Nashville, TN.
Distributed by APG Sales and Fulfillment, Nashville, TN;
    1-800-327-5113

WHAT EXPERTS ARE SAYING ABOUT
INSIDE ALZHEIMER'S

"...*Inside Alzheimer's* is a practical, conversational guide for those new to the disease, as well as advice and techniques for seasoned professionals...[This book] helps families and caregivers better understand individuals with Alzheimer's through love, acceptance, and communication."

— ForeWord Magazine

"*Inside Alzheimer's* provides evidence, through a variety of stories, that people with dementia are filled with possibilities for connection and meaning. Nancy Pearce provides both family and professional caregivers some valuable tips and strategies for hearing the person who has dementia. The stories will resonate with many readers and bring joy, tears, and increased awareness of the possibilities we each can bring in order to honor the person."

— *Jan Dougherty, RN, MS,* Director of Family and
Community Services Banner Alzheimer's Institute

"*Inside Alzheimer's* is beautifully written...in an easy to follow format...with examples and storytelling [that] make it very entertaining without taking away the insightfulness. Ms. Pearce gives a different dimension to the exhausting and very often overwhelming task [of providing] care...and shows that connection is possible, no matter how debilitated and compromised the person. The book, however, is beyond making connections with these persons—it is universal. In my opinion, the paradigms stated in the book are applicable to...all encounters we want to be meaningful. Wouldn't this world be a much happier place if we all intended true connections with each other? I will be recommending this book to everyone!!!"

— *Judith Davagnino, coauthor of* When Your Loved One
has Dementia: A Simple Guide for Caregivers

"*Inside Alzheimer's*...celebrates the hidden potential discovered when we consciously focus on the person's remaining abilities instead of his/her deficits. Through simple steps and inspiring case studies, Nancy demonstrates how we can all help persons with dementia transcend the seeming boundaries of the disease to experience profound moments of beauty, meaning, dignity, laughter and love.

— *Maribeth Gallagher,* Psychiatric Nurse Practitioner
Dementia Program Director, Hospice of the Valley

"Instead of reviewing...the repetitive information that many books provide, Ms. Pearce brings the reader to the root of understanding the individual...Using her basic concepts can change the face of care giving all together."

— *Gina M. Kastrup,* MSW Director of Social Services,
Riverside Health and Rehab. Center

To Ida Nadel (she was such a person!)

and to

Barbara and Maxine, her very special daughters

Table of Contents

Acknowledgments

This book has been over 50 years in the creating. It is the result of my process of listening and learning along, at times, a quite awkward life path—one that may not have been easy for those around me to witness. So many people have had great influence on my learning and have helped me to keep moving forward that I cannot possibly acknowledge each one of them in this brief text. There are several people in particular, however, who were inspirational, encouraging and supportive to me in the writing of this book.

With all my heart, I am deeply grateful for my loving family. My husband Bill has miraculously been able to flow with my shifting emotions, and has provided unswerving support and space when needed, hugs, dances and a constant loving presence. He and my sons are men who give me hope for the future because of their capacity and willingness to fully express tenderness and love. They have encouraged me to grow and reach far beyond what I ever thought possible. David, thank you for your graphic editing skills, the flowers and the sparkling excitement in your voice. Jason, thank you for your artistic sensibility, the laughter and the exquisite vibrations of Rachmaninoff, Liszt and Beethoven. I also want to thank Jan, my sister, who has beautifully expressed her celebration of my blossoming and who has perfected the art and sensitivity of blessed timing!

I give thanks to the many gifted healers and mentors who have helped expand my relationship with spiritual and creative realms. Barbara Collins and Pat Bolger have actively guided me to fully enter life, and each continues to deeply touch me with her sensitivities and sisterhood. Linda Keiser Mardis, Frédéric Lionel, and the Hana-Kai have energetically supported me on multiple levels and continue to expand my understandings of the power of connection. Thank you, Nancy Murray, for your unwavering friendship, the daily support of your poetry and for reminding me to use my left brain. Thank you Peg Reduker, for that beautiful expression of delight and joy—recalling it motivated and energized me as I began each morning. Thank you, Trisha Schlossberg, for the diversion when needed. I am also blessed to have had the daily support of the Blue Ridge Mountains and the sentiment rocks given to me by the remarkably caring staff at the Hospice and Palliative Care of Connecticut. To all these beautiful people who are geographically so far away, you are all fully present in my daily life and in my heart.

I want to express my appreciation to the dozens of people who over the past 20 years have shared their favorite resources with me—the most frequently mentioned are compiled in the Suggested Resources section at the end of this book. My profound gratitude goes out to the many reviewers who provided such wonderful feedback from the semi-polished draft of the book: Janet Johnston, Linda Keiser Mardis, Bill Gutermuth,

Trisha Schlossberg, Nancy Murray, Jack Gesino, Dr. Kay Davidson, Gina Kastrup and Barbara Collins. You have all helped to make this book honor persons with dementia and the caring individuals in each person's life. A special thanks also goes out to John Cole, the amazing Graphic Designer who created the cover design and typeset this book. Your steady guidance has made the process so much less scary and your enthusiastic participation has been a joy!

From the bottom of my heart, I want to thank two very dear friends and the main editors of this book, Judith Blahnik and Sharon Creal. They helped me to see my personal possibilities while supporting, cajoling and holding the faith. Judith was artfully able to encourage me to go deeper, inspire me with poetic wisdom, write gentle critiques that moved me forward and opened doors, and to enhance the clarity in wording and phrasing to make things POP. Sharon has continued to walk with me for so many years and displays such enthusiastic encouragement, clarity in vision and a delightful sense of humor. These two women are a writer's dream come true. Thank you both for helping to make this book clearer and more reader-friendly. Thank you for your precious presence in my life—you're the best!

Last and most importantly, I give my deepest gratitude to the countless persons with dementia and the families, friends and care professionals I have been privileged to meet and interact with over the years. The great many of you have been my finest teachers and greatest inspiration. You continue to live in my heart as I more fully practice how to share your wisdom and love with the rest of the world.

Preface

I'm here, in 'ere—I'm here, in 'ere!

Judy desperately shouted, "I'm here, in 'ere," every minute or two during the final hours of sunset. Every day she sat with others around the action of the nursing station in the late afternoons, but that didn't seem to help locate or comfort her—"I'm here, in 'ere" continued to pierce through everything else. Judy, who earlier in the day was laughing and blowing kisses, was now locked inside her devastating illness, calling out for someone to figure out how to find her, help her, be with her. For her, as is true for many, feeling isolated and locked out of the possibility of human connection was a predatory nightmare.

We—her care professionals, family and friends—also felt isolated and locked outside of her illness when we attempted to interact with Judy. As her disease progressed, our opportunities to relate with Judy lessened as any connected interactions with her became increasingly difficult and sometimes impossible. We grew frustrated by our inability to help Judy feel comforted; we missed her laughter and kisses. Eventually, we began to deem her out of reach and to look at her as the disease rather than the human being who, like the rest of us, needed exactly what we needed.

Just like me, Judy and other persons who have dementia need to feel a part of the flow of the intangible gifts of humor, wisdom and understanding found within the person-to-person connection. These needs can continue even through the end-of-life process. Unlike me, however, the person with dementia is often beyond remembering how to connect with others and can only relate as she is, here and now. Bridging a connection is up to me, up to us.

This book is written for anyone—care professionals, family members, friends and others—who desires to make meaningful connections with persons who have dementia. The path for encouraging the person with dementia to participate in life and human interactions lies in *our* opening to enter *her* world. When we are able to join the person in her world, we can see the many ways she continues to express her wisdom, or makes gestures that enfold us, or enjoys moments of mutual spontaneous emotion. When we share such experiences, each of us moves out of isolation and hopelessness. Each of us is empowered forward to grow—regardless of how far the disease has progressed.

Easing the isolation must begin and end with seeing the person with dementia as a *person*. In writing this book, I have deliberately avoided the objectified and generalized clustering of persons into *people-with-dementia*, victims trapped inside a web of difficult to manage symptoms and behaviors, or similar labels that explicitly or implicitly suggest that the person is no longer whole. Even in the unraveling of some dynamics, I have chosen to continue to discuss each topic with the use of personal pronouns of *his* or *her*, rather than *they* or *them,* to encourage the reader to become less academic and distanced and enter a more personalized connection with what is being said.

I have also chosen to use storytelling to place you, the reader, in rich, real-time interactions with persons who have dementia and to deemphasize the standard clinical, what-to-do approaches of Alzheimer's literature. Names and some personal details were changed to protect the person's and family's privacy, but the integrity of each story remains unchanged and pure. These are the persons who encouraged me to see inside the chaotic disease process and to open up to relating in a deeper, less inhibited, more authentic and heart-felt way. The evolution of each connection with each person helped my logic and my emotions make room for a new dimension of experience, a knowing on a very different level. Each story in this book is about a person with dementia guiding me to an opening where I could hear what she was saying— inside the broken words and frequently beyond the words—and discover a simple dependable practice of six basic human principles or concepts to use in bridging my way into connection.

My retelling of each person's story over the past 20 years, highlighting the use of one or more of the six concepts, has helped countless family members, friends and care professionals bridge the gap between their known, comfortable worlds and the sometimes daunting uncharted territory of time spent with the person who has dementia. In reading the stories, you may embark on an emotional journey. It is important to give yourself permission to read at your own pace. The more ways you can relate to the stories and the concepts presented, the greater your potential will be for making connections in general. Anyone can do it—it simply takes willing openness, some time…and patience. If you need help with practicing the concepts I present, there is a Working it Out section in each chapter that describes the exercises I do to stay in receptive, creative shape. Pick and choose what appeals to you or simply skip them to move on to the next chapter. There are no *should's* or *have-to's*. Be kind to yourself.

My hope is that the individual dynamism and beauty of each person I have connected with inside the dementia will astonish you, as they did me, and encourage you to interact with persons who have dementia with positive, possible and respectful regard. I encourage you to expand your sense of the possibilities and explore your own relationship with a person who has dementia. Help create connections that can be pleasurable, satisfying and even life-changing for you both. Open to discovering how each person's wisdom, as well as your own, will emerge.

How could anyone ever tell you
You were anything less than beautiful?
How could anyone ever tell you
You were less than whole?
How could anyone fail to notice
That your loving is a miracle?
How deeply you've connected to my soul!

A song written by Libby Roderick
From *The Hunger for Ecstasy*
Jalaja Bonheim, Ph.D., author
www.jalajabonheim.com

1 – Introduction

I suppose I jumped off the traditional academic path when I became disillusioned with armchair social theories in graduate school. It was the early 1970s and the country was seriously divided by racial tensions and war moratoriums. I chose sociological research, thinking my strong interest in discovering common understandings across cultures could make a difference in the current world; I thought there must be some bonding aspects among human beings as well as those which apparently drive us apart. But after that graduate year, much of which was spent exploring statistical analysis of sociological data, I wound up rather cynical, thinking anyone could prove practically anything with the creative manipulation of statistical data. By the time I graduated I was less interested in research and more passionate about getting into the "real world," to have concrete experiences and expose myself to new understandings.

During the next 15 years, I certainly did experience that real world! I married, had two sons and found myself working in jobs that were not usually considered open to women. I went from climbing telephone poles as an installer, to being foreman of an installation gang for the phone company, to renovating houses as a home improvements contractor. I loved the hands-on physical reality of my work. It energized me. The expectations were clear—just do the job. It felt good at the end of the day to step back and see that I accomplished something identifiable and concrete.

During the earlier years with the phone company, however, the mere presence of a woman, especially the only woman on the job, created anger in my co-workers. This confused and surprised me. I was the only woman in the country at the time being groomed for outside plant management. I thought that was a good thing, something to celebrate. I was a pioneer and I knew I was making it easier for other women to follow. In the meantime unfortunately, there were no other women to talk with about the isolation I felt, or about the disconnection from my co-workers and the painful judgments and accusations I heard every day.

There were a few courageous men on the job who bucked the peer pressure and attempted to relate to this new phenomenon— me. One man in particular initiated a conversation with me one day. He sincerely wanted to understand how I could see myself as a woman if I was doing a "man's job." I said that he and I had read different books on the subject of men, women and work. In my book I could do anything I wanted to do. I was young and not thinking according to the bias that had constrained my co-workers. I suggested to him that if his book says that a woman wears a skirt, sits at a desk, answers phones and by all means keeps her legs crossed all of the time, then that would make it very hard for him to imagine someone like me climbing telephone poles. To his credit, he eventually opened to accepting me as a woman and co-worker who really enjoyed and was good at the work. Few others had the courage to open their minds and change their thinking—most continued to clutch at their secure images and to, at best, keep me at a distance. Meanwhile, I wanted to be in the flow of relationship with those around me, to feel some form of connection, but there I was in an environment that pushed me to the side.

Later on, my job change to home improvements contracting allowed me to creatively expand on the hard work I enjoyed without the day-to-day absence of camaraderie and mutual respect. It required me to be in creative relationship with my clients. I came alive in the collaborative one on one brainstorming and planning to actualize a vision of a particular space or project with my clients. This shared part of the work invigorated me. I expanded when I listened to and understood my clients' ideas and experiences. Unfortunately, that time spent with the client was only a small portion of the work compared to the long hours I spent alone to complete each project. There it was again, that sense of isolation. It continued to gnaw at me until I became very clear about needing to learn how to create more of the connecting experiences that made me feel vital, grounded, inventive and receptive in my work and personal life.

I began to read just about anything I could get my hands on—from pop psychology to religious traditions—to understand more about the nature of my disconnection and the ways I could open myself to more connection. I went back to some old assigned readings from a comparative religion course I had taken 15 years earlier—back to the common threads that produce bonds or relationships among people. I reacquainted myself with the great monotheistic religions of Christianity, Judaism, and Islam as well as with Hinduism and Shamanism. I took a deeper look at Buddhism, Zoroastrianism, Confucianism and Taoism. I read modern day spiritual teachers and writings from a variety of indigenous religions.

A practice commonly mentioned in all of these spiritual traditions reminded me of something that I briefly experimented with during my years in college—the daily discipline of meditation or prayer. My hope was that the traditional teachings were accurate in their claims that a spiritual practice and a discipline of meditation or prayer would connect me first with my inner self, then with others in the world, and finally with a great field of energy that apparently envelopes all of us.

My renewed practice of meditation energized and surprised me. For one thing, I began to connect with the long-forgotten experience of being four years old and sitting with my mother after she injured her leg. I remembered putting my hands on her leg and knowing that we all have an ability to pass healing energy through our touch with loving consciousness. At four years old of course, my frame was more like, if I put my hands on the boo-boo it will make it feel better. This compelling and lingering memory, combined with my persistent need to heal my own perception of disconnection and coincidently several powerful experiences I had had with chronically ill friends all led me to study and train in a Japanese hands-on healing discipline called Reiki.

That's when the dreams began. Every morning I woke up with the same one about me being in a large room with chronically ill and dying people. My job was to be present with them through their process. Just that. My heart knew that this recurring dream was to be my life's work, but my mind fought it with a vengeance. After all, I had spent 15 years building a solid business. Both my sons were about to start school and I was ready to kick my business into full gear. More compelling and to the point, I *really* didn't want to go back into academia, which is exactly what this recurring dream would demand! After three months and three days of the same daily dream, my same self-torturous resistance to it, and the patient listening of friends and family throughout hours of my whining and mental squirming, I finally decided to return to school as a candidate for a master's degree in social work. That was the day the dreams stopped.

My social work education was excellent. I was well trained in assessing the biological, psychological, social, emotional and environmental influences on an individual's ability to function in the world. It was noticeable to me, however, that the social work literature up to the mid-80s showed little impetus to delve into the individual's spiritual beliefs and influences, which have since become the core of my own work. Still, I felt confident in the use of therapeutic interventions to help people move beyond their difficulties to balance and effective functioning in their world. The variety of theories and concepts were fascinating and I enjoyed bringing them to bear in my work with my clients.

During my second year, I interned at a large long-term care nursing facility. Here I thought was the perfect place to begin working with persons who were dying and to hone my skills as a clinician with persons who had chronic illnesses. My dream was about to take shape. But soon into that year, I found that I spent most of my time working with persons who had dementia and this presented one of those real-world unexpected problems.

Absolutely none of my training addressed how to work with persons who had dementia. The cognitive models were not very useful when I met a person whose cognition shifted from one moment to the next and whose ability to retain insights did not appear to exist.

What I did discover, though, was that I loved being with persons with dementia and it seemed that more often than not we were able to have a positive impact on each other. I would greet a person with mild to profound dementia at the front entrance of the facility and he would enthusiastically react to me as though I were a long-lost relative or friend. If a person's confusion led him into a fearful rage, I was able to listen to his concerns and help create a shift toward his feeling safe and better able to accept those moments. These persons were open, responsive, tender and beautifully appreciative of the simplest of gestures. I was hooked! I loved being with and working with each one!

Seriously, how could I have avoided falling in love with a woman like Anna who greeted me each time with "Oh, Lynnie! So wonderful to see you!" and reminisced about how we used to chase the boys when we were 17. And Mr. Miller! He was incapable of talking in any way that I could understand but came to life when he heard a waltz. He rose up to his full height and danced with great dignity and grace. And Sophie would laugh from her toes to her eyebrows, her entire body shaking in delight whenever I approached. Even though I understood this may not have been a compliment, I enjoyed being a part of the fun! My daily experience was telling me that these persons with dementia had something to give; each was helping me get in touch with a playfulness and joy I had long forgotten.

Other professionals and family members began to ask me what it is that I *do* to get persons with dementia to respond. My frustration began to grow when I realized I had no accessible answer. My heart or gut seemed to allow the person with dementia to guide me, and I would follow his lead. When I let him lead, I would come to know what to do or say. But I did not have a way to translate my behavior into a logical form to teach others. I could certainly give examples as to what to do in particular situations, yet each person is beautifully unique and requires an individualized approach. What strikes a chord for one person with dementia may not even begin the heart song for another. Twenty years later, I am still adding to the list of approaches that have been helpful in making connections—approaches that my clients have helped me learn. More to the point, I have discovered that it isn't so much about what I did or did not say or do that was key to pass on to professionals and family members—it was more about the way in which I was *being with* the persons who have dementia that seemed important to communicate. I thought there must be some basic, teachable concepts that would help others to understand and to realize the joys of being with these beautiful individuals.

IDA

Then Ida came into my life. As her daughter described her, "The prettiest smile, the most joyous laugh." So true! She just lit up the world of those who could really see her. Ida was still able to walk with some assistance, but her ability to put words together and to communicate thoughts had been severely compromised. Within a relatively brief time frame, her words were not able to be understood at all. Every verbalization was forced out with a strain, syllables mixed around into nonsensical sounds. Yet every attempt was filled with intent and passion. It felt as though whatever was being communicated must be very important to Ida. So, of course, it was important for someone to listen.

Each day I invited Ida to join me for a walk. We walked arm in arm through the nursing units on the second floor, the administration offices and back to her unit. All the while, Ida talked. Some days I could not understand any of her words and I learned to ask if what she was talking about was good news or bad news so as to respond appropriately throughout our walk. I would say, Ida, is that OK for you? She would either respond with shaking her head "Yes" and give one of her great smiles, or she would look at me as if I had just flown in from Orion. Whatever her response, I followed her lead. We would then proceed down the hallways with her talking away and with me periodically providing joyous responses or empathy and reassurances. Every day Ida was able, we walked the loop and talked. For almost two years this continued—each of us appreciating our time together yet I still understood neither the content nor the importance of her words nor why our walk and talk seemed so important to do. Then one day, during one of our walks, Ida stopped, turned fully towards me, held both of my arms, and said,

"I love you. You treat me like such a person!" She then turned and continued walking while speaking her nondiscernible language.

I was stunned. In that one moment, the two of us went beyond the nuts and bolts of ordinary communication—the frequently predictable patterns of statements and responses that move a conversation along between two people. Ida expressed that she felt that I was truly *seeing* her as a person during our interactions and in that moment I felt Ida was truly *seeing* me. We were two persons sharing a mutual experience of appreciation and validation for simply being ourselves. In that one moment, Ida taught me the importance of our time together. I realized then that what is helpful to anyone with dementia is to *connect with each as a PERSON*, rather than as someone with dementia, someone with a deficit, someone who is not whole.

Instead of focusing on working with persons who have dementia, therefore, my focus shifted toward understanding the essential aspects of how and why we connect with each other as persons. This, I thought, would help me more fully grasp what Ida was teaching me. I discovered some exciting literature on the nature of relationships and connection in the Stone Center Working Paper Series at Wellesley College, especially in the works of Dr. Jean Baker Miller, author of *Toward a New Psychology of Women* and co-author of *The Healing Connection*. According to Miller, a woman's sense of self and of worth is grounded in the ability to make and maintain relationships and that the most terrifying and destructive feeling that a person can experience is isolation, in the sense of feeling locked out of the possibility of human connection. Dr. Alexandra Kaplan in *Women's Growth in Connection* suggests that the basic human motive is the motive to participate in connection with others.

Who would more fully experience isolation and severe disconnection than a person with dementia? During one of her more confused days, Ida was sitting near the nursing station. She tried over and over again to get the attention of anyone in the flurry of people rushing by her. At first she smiled and tried to establish direct eye contact. Ida was clearly a woman who spent a lifetime in social connection with others and when the smile didn't work, she leaned over and grabbed at anyone passing by. Some people pulled away and continued on. Some scolded her. Then, of course she called out in her language of many noises. When no one responded she turned up the volume. Then people did respond, telling her to stop shouting and to keep quiet. Ida eventually retreated into herself with tears. What else could she do? She was powerless over changing her situation, helpless over connecting with others, essentially invisible.

Working with Ida and with other persons who have dementia taught me that my function was not to figure out what actions I could take to help her. It was not about her *getting* anything from me, or my *doing to* or *doing for* her. As Dr. Jean Baker Miller writes, *"it is about being in the flow of human connection rather than out of it."*

Persons with dementia helped me learn that the diagnosis of dementia does not, by itself, alter a person's enjoyment of or satisfaction with being in connection with others. The disease does, however, alter a person's ability to maintain connections, which poses challenges for those of us who are not sure how to connect when the rules change. By rules, I mean the familiar or predictable learned behaviors or ways of interacting that are generally accepted as socially appropriate. We can feel lost when we try to connect with a person who is not playing by the same rules from moment to moment. How do we relate to someone who doesn't speak with the same familiar sentence structure as we do or who uses the wrong words all the time? What are we supposed to do when the person with dementia comes to the party wearing her bra over her dress? What do we say when a 94-year-old woman thinks she is still raising young children that need to be picked up from school? How are we supposed to react when we have known this person our whole lives and she is not responding to us like she used to or, perhaps, does not even know us at all any more?

Connecting with the person who has dementia is challenging because he progressively forgets the rules for connection. Whatever his disease process, the person with dementia becomes decreasingly able to connect in familiar ways. This point cannot be overstated, by the way. In the widely read caregiver's standard, *The 36-Hour Day*, authors Nancy Mace and Peter Rabins remind us that the person with dementia is unable to remember and his unusual behaviors are a result of a disease process. It might be structural changes in the brain and/or destruction of brain tissue but something has occurred in the brain that has changed the person's ability to connect with others. His memory and behavioral problems are simply beyond his control...they are not chosen, not deliberate. We cannot expect the person with dementia will be able to adapt to our standards and rules.

This, of course, means that if a connection is going to occur, *it is up to us.* We will need to make the adjustments necessary to bridge the gap between ourselves and the person with dementia. The more I worked with caregivers and families, however, I discovered that frequently our attempts to connect with persons who have dementia can ignite our most hidden fears, insecurities and our deepest grief. These are significant barriers to participating in the flow of human connection. It became clear then that if I were ever to teach others about connecting with the person who has dementia I needed first to explore the ways we can get ourselves beyond these personal barriers and into the steps that help us construct bridges between each other. What are the ways in which we can more fully open to connecting with the person and to discovering the gifts he still has to offer?

I was living with this unanswered question when, in 1990, I attended a conference with a teacher of the Western Mystic tradition, Frédéric Lionel. Frédéric had an astounding mind and a stunning ability to conceptualize universal patterns and to see interrelationships among everything that exists. At the opening session, he stated that he was not there to teach us anything new—he was there to *remind us of what we already know and have forgotten.* In his lectures, I was reminded of the core elements that wisdom traditions have taught for eons about how to live in this world. And I knew that these core concepts were somehow a part of the bridge I was looking for, a part of the way toward understanding how we can open more fully to connecting with the person inside the dementia.

During a private consultation with Frédéric, I thanked him for reminding me of what I knew but had forgotten. He politely listened and then looked at me intently and said, "Yes, but how will you take action?" I had no clue, yet clearly, Frédéric threw the challenge out to me to go beyond remembering to taking real action that would create a positive change.

The challenge lit a fire in me and soon an action emerged. What surprised me was that my course of action did not come from me or Frédéric or any of the books I had been reading. It came from fifteen years of interactions with persons who have dementia. In those years at work, I paid attention—looking hard at my interactions with each person with dementia for the ways in which he had been affected by me, by others, and by the world even as he progressed through the disease. It is the person with dementia who guided me during all of the connections and disconnections toward identifying six basic concepts or principles that help bridge personal barriers and create genuine shared relationships. I have listed the concepts not in order of importance necessarily but in a way to create the easy to remember acronym, **IF LOST**:

Intend a connection
Free yourself of opinions/judgments/expectations
Love
Open to being loved
Silence
Thankfulness

These concepts or principles are the building blocks of the bridge between the ethereal and concrete aspects of being in connecting moments with persons who have dementia. They help translate what the heart knows into a logical, easy-to-understand form in the real outer world.

In the chapters that follow, I tell dozens of stories about connecting and relating to persons with mild to severe dementia. You will read how using the **IF LOST** principles can open your heart and expand your ability to permeate the fog that may seem to exist between you and the person with dementia. You will learn how to experience and share authentic moments of connecting and relating. Each chapter guides an exploration of one of the principles and reinforces your practice of the principle with simple suggested exercises.

I hope your journey into experiencing connections with persons who have dementia is filled with peaceful curiosity, gentle playfulness and exquisite openness. Let's get started.

2 - Intend a Connection

All major spiritual and wisdom traditions teach getting along with others—seeking unity rather than separation from one another and living in harmony. This peaceful state of being is not a mindless one, but one that we bring about by consciously taking actions. By *consciously*, I mean having an awareness of the power of our intentions. Popular authors like Deepak Chopra and Wayne Dyer helped raise a lot of interest in the possible effects of intention—that is, how the deliberate and clear focus of our thoughts and awareness may actually shape the world. As Michael and Justine Toms, cofounders of New Dimensions Radio, write, "Intention is the force that has the power to manifest what you want to happen."

If I have the intention—the deliberate and clear focus of thought and awareness—to establish a harmonious connection with a person who has dementia, it is more likely the connection will happen. When I say this to people who ask for help with better connecting with a person who has dementia, I hear a variety of reactions: "OF COURSE I intend to connect," someone will say, treating my point as a no-brainer, "but nothing I do works." Others abruptly cut to the chase saying, "Why else do you think I'm here listening to you!?!"

The fact is, most people I talk with do have the intention to connect, however what brings them to me is that something keeps getting in the way, something they say they cannot quite name. All they can tell me is that the connection is not happening. I encourage them to be willing to see and identify what might be getting in the way of connecting with the person who has dementia. Remarkably, to bring just a little attention to such barriers can be enough to allow them to shift and to clear a path for one's best intention to take shape. I put these barriers into two categories: the *Gremlins* and the *Presentation*.

In being with persons who have dementia, I have unearthed more of my personal gremlins than I knew existed and in turn discovered some gremlin-induced behaviors that betrayed my intentions and interfered with connections. Interestingly enough, and *because of* the disease process of the person with dementia, this discovery has not been painful or difficult for either of us. Very often the person does not have the memory of specific moments, including the nonconnecting moment I may have just fumbled. She simply may move into a different moment. I realized that when she is in a different place, with the next interaction I can be, too. When she lets go, I can do the same. We can both have a fresh beginning and I can feel joy in the freedom to simply be new with each interaction. This awareness has given me a sense of humor about my own gremlins, which in turn has helped me give myself permission to fail and to understand that tomorrow is another day and another opportunity to connect. I have learned to keep an open sense of peaceful curiosity and to maintain gentle playfulness.

THE GREMLINS

Gremlins are those persistent little thoughts that throw a wrench into the works and freeze everything up. They are the negative inner messages that stop you from doing anything you are trying to do. If you are like most people, you come fully equipped with all the *shoulds*, *oughts* and insecurities that your personal psychology and society has to offer. And gremlins remind you of them day and night. You want to make a connection with someone? It just will not happen as long as you pay attention to their messages. Your gremlin's job is to distract you from and to interfere with that connection.

I guarantee that it will not take long to identify your own gremlins as you attempt connections with persons who have dementia. The disease process does not destroy a person's ability to feel all positive and negative emotions. Interactions tend to be very real and direct—at times, bluntly honest. Your sense of humor and a little humility will help you develop grace and ease in dealing with whichever gremlins surface.

Give Your Gremlin A Coffee Break

GLORIA

Gloria was a client who was able to live in her own home long after the onset of dementia. She had an extraordinary family; four children took turns providing continual supervision and care. My responsibility and pleasure was to regularly spend time with Gloria and encourage her reflections about her life whenever she was able to participate. On one particular visit, I arrived, my head spinning with all that I still needed to do that day. Not only had I been running to keep appointments, but there were four other persons still on the schedule, paperwork I did not even want to think about, and I had just been notified of a friend's personal crisis.

However, I wanted and intended to spend focused time with Gloria. I consciously worked hard at letting go of all the gremlin messages about what else I *should be doing* so I could be fully present with her. I remember thinking I had done a pretty good job of dismissing the negative and focusing on my intention. Apparently not. About ten minutes into our visit, Gloria pulled my face toward her with both hands on my cheeks, stared deeply into my eyes as though aiming for my heart, and said with a hauntingly painful plea, "*MEeee!*" Gloria was bringing my attention back to her, to where it belonged in that moment. My mind was somewhere else and she knew it.

A person with dementia tends to have very strong antennae; she can feel when we are distracted or are not fully present for a connection. She will sense when your gremlins are dividing your attention, quite possibly even though you are not aware of it. If you pay attention, you will see the signs of your preoccupation in the person's reactions. It may be as easy to understand as Gloria's reaction or it may be nonverbal in an irritated look, fidgeting, or pushing your hand away. At minimum, a connection between the two of you will not happen in those moments.

Gremlins have a variety of messages that botch things up. I will talk about some of the more common ones, but first I would like to reassure you. Some of us have very strong relationships with our gremlins, so I will not suggest that you ban them from your life. I only suggest that you give your gremlin a little coffee break during the time you want to spend in connection with the person who has dementia—just for that time. It will allow you to be fully, really, and honestly present in that moment and to bring your full attention to connecting. Do not worry. Your gremlins will eagerly come back when you are done. So let's talk about some of those messages.

Oh That Poor, Unfortunate Soul

One of the fastest routes to making no connection at all is pity. As Caroline Myss so aptly points out in her *Essential Guide for Healers*, you cannot be effective if you can only look at a person and see the tragedy, the horror, the sadness. To pity someone with dementia is to see her only through her illness, her diagnosis. It places a distance between the two of you with you on a better-than-the-other level. Pity's only function is to keep you in a sad place and the person with dementia beyond reach. A harmonious connection requires the two of you to be on the same playing field. Each of you is a person who has something valuable to offer in a relationship and each of you will be better for having connected with the other.

Pity also promotes despair—hopelessness about ever escaping the condition. On the other hand, seeing a person with dementia as someone who is going through an experience that demands some difficult adjustments, empowers both of you and provides a direction. There are tools to learn and skills to develop that will help both of you as you adjust to changes as they occur. This is doable. It promotes strength and hope.

MARY

I did not think that pity was a gremlin I needed to work on, since such a large focus of mine as a medical social worker has been to empower my clients. Then Mary came into my life to teach me more. I visited Mary in her nursing facility every few weeks over a period of five months. Her norm was to be in a searching mode—something was not quite right. She had difficulty finding words to express herself, and she experienced many moments of frustration and anxiety that were not easily shifted. I spent my time pushing her in her wheel chair around the facility to assist in her search, all the while talking in soothing tones. She would occasionally dip into a very painful past and dart away with an abrupt shift in topic or direction for our tour. The visits always ended with my validating her connection with her daughter—"the only person that ever really loved me," she would say. Our time together helped calm her for a few hours, sometimes for a few days. Unfortunately, she would always return to that anxious, searching place.

During one visit, shortly before she died, Mary had an amazingly clear day. She talked with only slight word-finding difficulty about multiple tragedies throughout her life. Her story gripped me. She revealed her history of abuse, of people who had abandoned her, and of her feelings of inadequacy and failure. I became almost overwhelmed with sadness, feeling sorry for *this poor, unfortunate soul* who had such a difficult path in life. Tears began to well up in my eyes, I must admit.

Then I noticed that Mary was speaking in a matter-of-fact way. She had no tears, no particular emotions associated with such traumatic events and no detachment either. All appeared to be integrated and she was at peace with everything. Her serenity made me wonder about my welling-up sadness even while she so clearly communicated from a position of strength. I asked her how she was able to adjust so beautifully to all the things that had happened to her in this lifetime. She straightened up her frail, 86-year-old frame and said, "Well, honey, if you can't adjust in this world, you're just shit out of luck!" I laughed and immediately felt lighter and stronger. I let go of the pity that had put me in tears and identified with Mary's strength and humor. We created a new bond that day and we were actually able to embrace, which was something Mary had not been capable of before.

Certainly, it is valuable to empathize with the person who has dementia and to put yourself in her shoes so that you can understand and have compassion for what she is experiencing.

Then, you, as a person, are identifying with her as a person. When you pity, you are identifying with a myriad of symptoms and/or events, not the person. Empathy identifies with the person; pity identifies with the symptoms. Empathy places you on a level, person-to-person position, so you can work together in moments of healing connection and move forward.

Run For The Hills!!!

This gremlin says that there is something to fear in the connection. Fear, in its many forms, is one of the reactions that prevents people from opening to connecting with the person who has dementia.

LEE and ALICE

Lee and Alice lived on the same unit of a nursing facility. Both were in their late 70's and dementia prevented them from doing anything independently or from having simple interactions with others. Yet, Lee and Alice had each other. Every morning the staff did a wonderful job of getting both women ready for the day—clean dresses, jewelry and just the right amount of makeup; appearance had been very important to both of them throughout their lives. Every afternoon, Lee and Alice sat next to each other near the nursing station and chatted away. They looked at the hallway wall, which was blank—as we saw it. "Oh! What lovely flowers!" Lee would say. Alice would then look over at Lee and say something like, "Oh, yes! Extraordinary colors! Can you believe how beautiful?!" One or the other of them often used a word that made little or no sense. There were many times that the sentences were incomplete or formed in an unusual way. Nonetheless, whatever one said, the other accepted in a socially appropriate way and continued to move the dialogue forward.

This interaction typically went back and forth for over half an hour. Often, the dialogue was repeated as the day went on. Both women thoroughly enjoyed their connection and we thoroughly enjoyed witnessing it.

There were many days, however, that Lee needed to remain in bed. On those days Alice was lost. She sat near the nursing station, tearful and very distraught, but unable to verbalize the reason why. It did not help for us to explain that her friend was not feeling well or even to show her Lee in her room; Alice had no memory of the relationship from day to day, and Lee could not participate in the same way on her off days.

In an interdisciplinary unit team meeting, many staff identified that Alice missed and needed the type of exchange she had with Lee, which gave her joy and set her up for a great afternoon. We began to problem-solve about how to help Alice. It would be great, we thought, to have different staff members engage in similar dialogues with Alice in Lee's absence.

The fears then readily jumped to the surface: *I'm not crazy! I'm not going to talk to anyone about something that isn't there! I don't think I can do it. I wouldn't know what to say or do. Everyone will laugh at me; I'll never hear the end of it! I'm certainly not going to support their delusion; I'm here to orient them to reality* (more about that last one in the next chapter!).

Initially it can be a bit disconcerting to enter into a dialogue when you do not know the rules. Take a look, if you would, at the following cartoon:

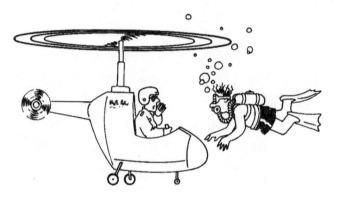

"I said: one of us is hallucinating!"

Copyright 1996 by Patrick Hardin

Can you honestly say you would not be a bit "weirded out" if you were either of those two people? The world as each of them thinks they know it is turned upside-down in that moment. In perhaps a less dramatic way, the feelings evoked when trying to connect with a person who has dementia can be similar. The sentence structure is not familiar to you; the words do not often make sense in the context; the focus of attention appears to shift randomly to different time frames. You are thinking about entering into someone else's uncharted territory. Your gremlin might tell you this is just too scary and you might withdraw or run or make yourself busy with other things. However, you could also choose to have your gremlin take a coffee break and see this as an amazing and exciting opportunity for an adventure.

There were a courageous few, at first, who were willing to give their fear gremlins a coffee break and explore the adventure of connecting with Alice. One nursing assistant in particular improvised freely and loved what she called those *just-us-girls-hanging-out* moments. We all saw how playfulness created effective connections that were helping Alice have a good day. Eventually, as more and more staff played along, we also saw a sense of competence and spirited camaraderie emerge within the whole unit!

Some fear gremlins do not easily take time off. We can be very attached to our territories—our sanity, our knowing and our own personal delusions. We tend to be very reluctant to do anything that has us question ourselves or that allows an opening for others to question us. The next chapter will discuss these attachments in more detail. In addition, there are some suggestions at the end of this chapter on releasing and letting go. I do know that if you can release the fear, even in those moments, the rewards will exceed the risk by far!

How Sad.
Remember How She Used To Be?

FRIEDA

Not such an easy one to release, even for brief times, this gremlin's message can feel so tender, at times it is like an old friend reminiscing with you. I vividly remember a talk with Frieda, the daughter of one of the residents at a facility. She was frustrated because she did not know what her mother was saying, how to be with her or how to respond. She passionately wanted to connect with her mother and she expressed deep sadness and pain with the disconnection. I listened, allowing her to vent her feelings and concerns. When she finally asked me how she could reach her mother, I moved right into teaching mode to provide her with concrete tools for relating with her confused mother. Frieda was attentive as she listened to me, nodding her head at all the appropriate moments. I felt very pleased to be helping her. "But I do not want to connect with this mother," she said gently when I finished speaking. "I want my mother back!"

I am thankful to Frieda for so clearly expressing the grief that can interfere with a family member's ability to connect with her confused loved one. To be fully open to connecting with her mother in the present, Frieda had to deal with the reality that the mother who raised and nurtured her, who gave strength to her and who always knew the right thing to do to put Frieda back on top of the world, was no longer available in the same ways. Frieda needed to focus on the need to grieve the loss of those and other aspects of the mother she missed. Once she began to acknowledge and work through some of her grief, she was able to release her longing for aspects of her mother that were no longer available and open at each visit to a real connection with her mother in current time.

The need to enter the grieving process is not the exclusive turf of the family. You may be a friend or a professional caregiver who had a particularly unique relationship with the person who has dementia. With each change in the person's cognition, her ability to interact with you in familiar ways shifts and you will experience a sense of loss. Our tasks are to remain aware of how these shifts affect us, allow the feelings to surface and open ourselves to moving forward through the grieving process. If you or someone in your life is having difficulty or feeling stuck, I recommend seeking out a trained professional social worker, counselor or other helping professional who specializes in grief counseling. They are worth it!

You Don't Really Want To Mess With This, Do You?

This gremlin supports your impatience, intolerance, irritation, defeat, disappointment and whatever other feelings make you resistant to pursuing a connection with a particular person. After all, connecting with a person who has dementia takes time and patience—that is a given. There will be days when your time and patience are low or when the person with dementia is having a very bad day, and her disease process may be preventing her from responding or interacting at all. To be honest, there will also be days when the person with dementia is just plain not pleasant to be around.

DORIS

At age 92, Doris had moderate dementia. My year of internship at her skilled care facility was Doris' third year living there. She hated being there and she hated the thought of becoming like "all these old and decrepit, senile and useless people." Her world consisted of her private room where she spent the day behind the closed door. At meal time, she came out but spoke to no one; she wore a frozen scowl on her face and scurried right back to her room after eating. She described the few people in her life—the staff and several distanced nieces and nephews—as irritating, insensitive and uncaring about her pain. In fact, the staff and her family were totally frustrated with Doris' constant complaining and her refusal to accept help. It was "nothing short of torture," her niece said one day, "to call on the phone and then have to hear a litany of gripes and complaints about life."

My supervisor assigned Doris to my student caseload—a wisdom I did not totally appreciate at the time! Week after week I listened to Doris' objections—the gossiping old ladies, aches and pains, selfish family, failing vision.

There was nothing good in her life and she did not mind rifling out the specifics over and over again. I tried to help her reframe situations, to refocus and to problem-solve solutions with all of my well-learned social work skills. The effort was futile and my gremlins continually harassed me: *Not even a saint could have the patience to sit with this woman! Man…this is just a waste of time! Maybe you aren't such a good social worker, Nancy.*

I really did not want to mess with Doris. Nothing seemed to be likeable about this old lady. The only thing I thought must be serving some purpose was my willingness to sit with her through her expressions of pain. So I kept returning. Besides, I had to; she was assigned to me!

After many hours and many weeks, I stumbled into a different awareness. I mean literally: I entered her room and tripped over my own feet. This being a frequent occurrence in my life, I have long-since learned to withhold embarrassment and go for the big finish with a musical "Ta-dahh." Doris stared at me for a moment and then just could not avoid that little up-turn to the corner of her mouth as she said, "Well, aren't you the clumsy ox!" That was Doris' slip! She showed me that she had a sense of humor—caustic of course, but a sense of humor nonetheless! We had a new beginning. I could relate to *that*!

During the months that followed, I still spent plenty of time listening to her complaints yet I could use humor in various forms to help budge her perspective. At a team meeting, I told staff about Doris' sense of humor—of course, who'd believe it, right? One nursing assistant believed me and approached Doris the next day when she came out of her room with me on what she called her Virgin Vacation Voyage. He gave her a great smirky smile and with his hands on his hips exclaimed, "My goodness! What did she have to pay you to get you out of that room?" Doris smiled, winked and quipped, "I don't remember, but you better believe it was a pretty penny!" Over time, Doris complained less, reported less pain and ended her isolation by establishing and reestablishing connections with others around her.

Doris was one of my greatest teachers. She was probably my biggest challenge in trying to make a connection, and yet I learned so much from staying with her. In my difficulties with entering her room each week, I had my first "in my face" awareness of my gremlin telling me that I did not really want to mess with this. Because she was on my assignment and I had to hang in there, I discovered the effectiveness of giving my gremlin a coffee break and reminding myself that I really *do* have the intention of connecting with this person.

Doris taught me that there is a loveable strength in the most feisty and ornery of persons. It is a strength that will transform both me and the person who has dementia when I reflect that strength back to her. I learned to remind myself to keep my heart and mind open to search for some aspect of the person that I can appreciate, enjoy, honor—any strengths she may have, anything positive to connect with. The quest for some aspect of a person you can truly like, admire and respect is an essential aspect of establishing a harmonious connection. The connection needs to feel good for both of you. The person with dementia has very strong antennae and will, on a very real level, know you are enjoying the interactions and connection. That will be the greatest gift for you both.

You Really Should Be More

Some people understandably feel frustrated when they try to connect; if a connection does not happen, their underlying feelings of inadequacy and failure can flare up: *I should be a more patient person. I should be able to figure out how to reach her.* To hold onto these messages will only continue to keep that barrier between the two of you because you're too busy listening to your gremlin verbally whipping you to listen to the person with dementia.

MRS. WILSON

Mrs. Wilson was 72 years old and multiple strokes had dramatically limited her abilities to both process information and express her thoughts clearly. Her inability to care for herself brought her to the skilled nursing home where I worked. Mrs. Wilson enjoyed sitting out with other people and spending her days waving, smiling and blowing kisses to everyone walking by. As you can imagine, we walked by her often!

One day, however, Mrs. Wilson was frantic. For half an hour every staff member on her unit tried to decipher what she was upset about. By the time I got there, everyone was as frustrated and upset as Mrs. Wilson. Her nursing assistant, who was sitting with her and holding her hand, gave me a summary of events. Then she tearfully said, "I should be able to figure out what she is saying." Suddenly, everyone began talking over each other, rushing into their stories of how they should have been able to understand. Above the cacophony, Mrs. Wilson's voice broke through, very clearly, "DON'T SHOULD ON YOURSELF!"

A long and total silence followed.

Mrs. Wilson scanned our faces and suddenly broke out laughing at our expressions, at the double meaning of her statement, at the joy of clearly expressing herself, at probably so many things. We laughed, hugged and completely shared the joy of that moment. The laughter helped us to loosen up, release, relax and open our hearts to each other. What a powerful connection we all made in that moment. We then took Mrs. Wilson's suggestion and gave that gremlin some time off. We could open again to being fully present to listen to her concern. Somewhere amid the releasing of tension, the experiencing of connection and the opening of our hearts to a fresh beginning, we deciphered what Mrs. Wilson was communicating. A few minutes later, watching her enjoy the cup of chocolate ice cream she had been asking for was pure joy for us all. We also brought away with us a great tool for countering that *should* gremlin with a touch of humor.

You Can't Do This. This Is Too Hard.

I'm going to confront this gremlin head-on: OF COURSE you can do this! Connecting with a person who has dementia is not rocket science. This is not too hard for you. You may need to develop a few new skills and, perhaps, awarenesses but your opening to connection will evolve with the holding of that intention and with the willingness to just relax and keep a sense of wonder for whatever unfolds. It is important to remember that *this is not about you! It is about how the two of you can connect, person to person.*

Many of us hear *You can't do this* when we are really disappointed because we see no signs of a connection happening. This is particularly common before the first experience of a powerful connection with a person who has dementia. It's normal to feel disappointed; you wanted that connection! However, I encourage you not to turn that disappointment into a belief that you cannot possibly make a connection with anyone who has dementia—ever. The lack of connection may be because it is simply not going to happen at this time. Remember that the person's ability to connect vacillates from moment to moment with this disease. It's OK to give yourself permission to get some space and regroup. At some point in the future, you can return with a fresh new intention and openness. At that time, the person with dementia may be more able to enter a connection.

The potential for connection always exists—in every human interaction. The person is still there, regardless of how advanced her dementia and how limited her ability to respond. She can still feel your presence and your willingness to connect with her.

You may only notice that her respirations calm down and become more even. Perhaps her contracted arms relax a bit or her rocking motions slow down or cease. Maybe her pale cheeks become more pink. These are all signs that your presence has affected her positively; you have connected with her in a way that provides her with comfort on probably more levels than you can know. This feels good for both of you. I guarantee that you will find successes that inspire you to continue to take the time.

Pay Attention To This Message: *You Can't Do This Any More!*

It is extremely important to know when you have had enough. The message, *You can't do this any more* implies that you have reached your saturation point over time; you're just plain burned-out, fried and done. If this is true, these words are most likely an inner wisdom telling you that some form of change must occur for *your* welfare and/or survival.

On a smaller scale, my initial difficulties in connecting with Doris, who constantly complained, taught me how important it is to remain vigilant over my frustrations. When I cannot let go of my frustrations during a visit and I begin to think *I can't do this any more,* for whatever reason, my *Temptee-Timer* equivalent pops up. The *Temptee-Timer* is that little plastic button in some turkeys that pops up when the turkey is done. It is the association I have when I finally understand that the interaction is not going anywhere, the connection is not happening now, and I am getting frustrated. When my inner *Temptee-Timer* pops up, I'm done. When that happens, I thank the person with dementia for allowing me to spend time with her; I say good-bye and let her know either when I will be back or certainly *that* I am coming back. I do this, by the way, whether or not I think what I'm saying *computes* for the person. The potential for understanding is always present.

I encourage you to listen to yourself and your inner wisdom to know when you have reached your saturation point during a particular interaction. It is very important to listen to your own needs in this connection, too. Once again, it needs to work for both of you.

On a larger scale, *You can't do this any more* may be your inner wisdom helping you understand that you are on overload. For example, you may have assumed, willingly or reluctantly, all of the care providing responsibilities, which may have expanded beyond what is possible for one person to accomplish. You may be spending too many hours each day providing care and giving up too many things that were very important to you before the person's disease progressed. You probably do not have enough hours in a day to get it all done, to get enough sleep, to even see straight. You may be totally burned out. If these are the kinds of reasons you hear *You can't do this any more, LISTEN*!!! Listen to your inner wisdom. It is definitely time to make a change.

If you have even the beginnings of awareness that you are becoming overwhelmed, it is beyond the time to problem-solve toward a more balanced plan of care. It is beyond the time to consider the welfare of everyone involved—the person who has dementia, all care people, and *you*! Consistency in care is impor-tant, but that does not mean that you are the only one who can provide great, consistent care for the person with dementia. You are not doing yourself or the person with dementia any favors when you are feeling impatient and exhausted. As confused as the person may be, she can still feel those barriers and the distancing. She can still, on some level, sense tension and stress in her environment even when she cannot verbalize or make sense of it.

If you are a family member feeling overwhelmed by the demands of being a care person, it is helpful—particularly when you are not seeing too straight at the time—to get together with care professionals and/or with other extended family members and friends and brainstorm some possible solutions to the stressful situation. Your local Alzheimer's Association is a wonderful resource and only a phone call away. Social workers and counselors who specialize in working with persons who have dementia are also wonderful resources to help provide some suggestions and creative alternatives. I am continually a witness to the care person's surprise at their family and friends pulling together with concrete actions that make the care person feel supported and provide concrete assistance.

If you are an overwhelmed care professional, it is time to brainstorm with your employer about alternatives to the currently stressful situation. Perhaps you can temporarily switch assignments with another professional to give yourself a break. Perhaps you need to be permanently reassigned. Perhaps venting your frustrations to another member of the care team and to have those feelings validated is enough to release some of that pressure that has been building up. The point is that it is definitely time to make a change of some sort for everyone's benefit.

PRESENTATION, PRESENTATION, PRESENTATION

You may find that you do not have any gremlins that are distracting you from connecting with the person who has dementia. Congratulations! You are one of the precious few, I must say. Yet, you sense there is something else standing between you and the person. Or you might be someone who finds that even with your diligent awareness and a good practice of sending your gremlins for coffee breaks, something is still interfering with your intention to connect with the person who has dementia. In either case I suggest you consider how you present yourself—meaning, how you communicate. I have heard it said that communication is 60 % body language, 30 % tone of voice, and only 10% the actual words. Whatever the statistics, communications experts tell us that the vast majority of communication has little to do with the words that come out of our mouths. It has almost everything to do with the way the words are presented. If we remain unaware of how we present ourselves, we may be setting up our well-intended connections for a very bumpy ride.

Sitting a moment and thinking about our own interactions in the world will tell us that this is so. When someone rushes toward us, hands on hips, wearing a frowning expression, we most likely become tense and prepare for some form of confrontation. We may be particularly sensitive to a loud, brash vocal quality or despise a high, squeaky voice. Perhaps the smell of a particular perfume is overwhelming or reminds you of a person from your past that you just could not stand. Sometimes a person you talk with is standing uncomfortably close, "in your face," or so far away she appears to not really want to be there. At times, you are not even able to identify why it is you react positively or negatively to another person, but the feeling remains very real.

A person with dementia has the same perceptions and takes in the same signals as her senses allow. She can feel our tensions, distractions or apathy because these are broadcast across our faces and in our body stances and voices. As the disease progresses, however, persons who have dementia become less able to find the words or to draw together concepts that help make sense of why the interaction with another person either does or does not feel right. As the disease progresses, she becomes less able to take in and understand the meaning of the words from others and becomes more dependent on our tone of voice and our body language to get a sense of what we are trying to communicate. Also as the disease progresses, she tends to have increasingly pure, uninhibited, honest emotions and positive and negative reactions to what she perceives. Even persons who have very progressed dementia and are essentially nonverbal and bed-ridden are responsive in ways we can observe, if we look closely. With the intention of establishing a harmonious connection with a person who has dementia, therefore, a deliberate focus of our attention needs to be brought to how we can present ourselves as persons who are open to that connection.

Before approaching the person with dementia, a very basic beginning point is to spend a few seconds and take a self-inventory. Bring your attention to where your thoughts are in that moment. Are you worrying about your bills or trying to figure out how you are going to get one child to her soccer game and the other to T-ball practice? Is that laundry list of everything you have to get done today just cranking away in your mind and driving you crazy? Now bring your attention to your body to see where you might be holding tension. Did you just stub your toe and feel LOTS of pain? Are your shoulders up around your ears? Are the muscles in your face tightened and your jaws powerfully clenched? Are you moving at light speed? *Please...give yourself a moment to just relax!* This is not healthy for you and it is a perfect setup for failure in relating to others.

Take a moment to breathe deeply and to try to allow past and future concerns or worries to flow out of your body. As you breathe, bring your attention to various parts of your body to "take a reading." Where you read tension, try allowing the tension to slip away with the exhaling of your breath. Bring your full attention to this, allowing all other thoughts to slip away with the exhaling of your breath. Slow down. Become fully aware of yourself in that moment.

Working with persons who have dementia has been one of the greatest gifts I have received because each has taught me, in her own way, the importance of relaxing into being in the present moment. Her only certain reality is in the present moment. That moment may be perceived by her to be in a different place or time, but it is her very real and present moment. The times I am maximally effective in relating to a person with dementia are when I have been able to let go of my perception of the world—worries, tensions, and concerns—and to join her in her present moment, wherever or whenever that may be.

Taking a moment to relax and bring yourself into the present will be directly reflected in your presentation to the person with dementia. You will have more of a calm, gentle approach.

Your voice will be more soft and soothing. You will approach in a slower, nonthreatening manner. You will be more open to spending time connecting with the beautiful person who is there and your body stance and voice will reflect that openness. You have just given both yourself and the possibility for a connection with the person who has dementia a very solid beginning.

SUMMARY

The most powerful action toward establishing a harmonious connection with a person who has dementia may be your holding the intention to do so. You will find increasing evidence of success when you bring a deliberate and clear focus of your thoughts to connecting person-to-person. As you do so, you will need to gently let go of whatever may be preventing you from feeling open and able to fully live in that moment. I encourage you to take some time to sit down in a relaxing, comfortable, quiet space and listen very carefully to see if you have any little gremlins that have been talking to you before, during, or after those moments of trying to connect with the person who has dementia. This certainly does not have to be a major trip into your subconscious by the way; who has the energy for that?! If you do, however, discover one or a few, just observe them without guilt trips or heavy *mea culpas*. Then practice letting them go; give them a coffee break. The purpose of the exercise is not to become self absorbed but to release those messages that can keep you from fully opening to connecting with the person who has dementia. Being aware of them or naming them is often enough to release their hold on you.

I also encourage you to take a moment before entering the space of the person with dementia to just breathe (see breathing exercise at the end of this chapter). While breathing, acknowledge your thoughts or worries and allow them to hitch a ride out with the exhaling of each breath. Pay attention to where your body may be holding on to tensions and allow the tightness to flow out of your body with each exhale. Since your intention is to connect, consciously make the adjustment to be fully open and present in the moment with the person who has dementia. Remember what Mary said: "If you can't adjust in this world, you're just shit out of luck!" What I do know is that with the adjusting—the conscious release of gremlins and whatever else separates us—comes a new openness and a new ability to connect harmoniously with the person who has dementia. With those moments of connection come joy, delight and playfulness. As you experience more and more of those moments, you will find that your patience will grow along with your ability to see and validate the minutest signs of connection.

The focus is on keeping ourselves as open as possible to being in the flow of person-to-person connection. Treating someone like a person means that we are fully open to interacting with her without fears, hesitations or attitudes. Treating someone like a person means that we respect that she has a full history, is wonderfully unique and is very worthy of getting to know. Treating someone like a person means that we are willing to take the time to interact with her with non-judgmental attentiveness.

WORKING IT OUT

*Live in the moment and create a feeling
of openness.*

Breathe it Out

Do this exercise any time or place for an immediate grounding effect. It will relax you and help shift your attention to the present moment, regardless of whatever distractions exist. Give yourself permission to set aside judgments about how well you are doing the exercise. Simply observe the comforting rhythm of your breathing.

Focus only on your breath as you inhale and exhale, taking perhaps four or five full seconds for each. As you breathe in, allow your breath to go deeply and easily down into your belly or diaphragm—the area below your rib cage. As you breathe out, allow all the air to escape. As you breathe in, feel the air expanding your lungs and stretching them out as if they were balloons filling, breaking up any tensions that may be present. As you breathe out, release any tensions in your body with the breath. As you breathe in, silently say the word "comfort;" as you breathe out, silently say the word "relax." Repeat as often as desired.

The Self-Hug

Place one of your hands over your heart and the other over your diaphragm and solar plexus, the area below your rib cage.

In tense or stressful moments, the heart rate becomes rapid and breathing is short and shallow. Placing your hands in these positions focuses your intention to calm and deepen the rhythms of each.

NOTE: this may be difficult to do discreetly in public— people could see you holding your hand over your heart and assume that you are having a heart attack! The solar plexus is usually easier to "hug" in less obvious ways. While sitting, it is very easy and looks quite comfortable to place one hand on top of the other as it rests over that area. Try different positions, explore it a bit, have fun with it. You will be amazed at how supportive it feels, when support is what you need most.

Phrases that Help Us "Let Go"

Certain expressions can encourage the release of obstacles that keep us separate from others. I already mentioned Mrs. Wilson's **"Don't should on yourself."** Another classic is: **"What other people think of me is none of my business."** A less well known expression is one that Sadie used. Sadie was born in Armenia in the early 1900s, lived through five wars, and saw "too much fighting, too much war." She witnessed and was the victim of "so much ugliness in this world" and yet even in her last days of life, when she was barely able to talk, she constantly blew kisses and silently mouthed the words "I love you" to everyone who entered her room.

I asked her daughter what Sadie's secret was that she had survived so much and remained open and loving. Her daughter said that the greatest lesson her mother taught her in life was to, **"Throw the glass of water over your shoulder."** This was not meant to be done literally, she explained. "If you find yourself faced with a conflict and you know that your heart is pure and you have no malicious intent, throw your concerns over your shoulder like a glass of water; pick up your chin and move forward into the world with a peaceful heart." Practice the art of letting go of your concerns, those little gremlins, and move forward toward connection.

Stretch it Out

The body holds tension unless we consciously release it. My tension is most often in my shoulders and neck. I frequently have to take time out during a busy day to bring my shoulders down from up around my ears and to stretch those muscles out. Take a reading of your body and find your own personal tension-holding place(s) and keep in mind the importance of helping those muscles stay limber to prevent seizing. Obviously, do not do any exercises or stretches that are not medically in your best interest. If you are not sure, ask your doctor.

The chest muscles commonly tense up under stress. When that happens, most of us feel tightness or constriction in the chest, as our heart races and our breathing becomes more rapid. This stretch takes a few seconds but it releases that feeling of tightness.

Place your hands on the small of your back, with palms touching the back in whatever position is comfortable. Now tilt your head gently backward so that you are looking upward (no need to force it—and don't tilt your head back if it causes you to be dizzy or faint). You will feel a slight pulling or stretching of the skin and muscles of the front of your neck and chest. Now gently pull back your elbows as if to have them touch behind your back. Do this just enough to feel a slight pulling or stretching of the skin and muscles across the front of your chest. Bring your full attention to the feeling of release from tension and the feeling of spaciousness or openness that this stretching generates.

3 – Free Yourself of Opinions and Judgments

While gremlins tug at our hearts and distract us with their messages, they can also activate long-held personal opinions and judgments about the world, ourselves and others. These form the mind-sets from which we make assumptions and often establish a course of action without open inquiry. They keep us from asking what else might be going on in the moment, either for the person with dementia or between the two of us. If we question our own opinions and judgments once in a while, we get a glimpse of how these habits of thinking can readily blame the shortcomings of the person with dementia rather than the ways in which we may be participating in a missed connection.

Although mind-sets interfere with our connecting with others, we strongly resist changing them. The philosopher Frédéric Lionel said, "Man would rather burn his house down than give up his opinions." I am certainly not going to suggest you burn your house down or go through any gut-wrenching changes in this chapter. I do encourage your openness to discovering and relaxing some of the strongly-held opinions and judgments you have regarding how to enter and proceed in the world.

Many religious and wisdom traditions lean heavily on threats of punishment for judging others harshly. That idea and practice tends to make me a bit defensive. At their best, such teachings strongly suggest that we withhold harsh judgment of others and instead look at our own imperfections and faults.

Frédéric opens this discussion with the statement, *"Dare* to be free of your opinions and judgments." This awakens my sense of challenge. If I take the dare, I can discover and release my hold on my opinions and judgments with a spirit of exploration and playfulness. I don't need to judge myself harshly; there are no dire consequences. It becomes a hide-and-seek type of game to uncover beliefs and attitudes that interfere with my ability to connect with the person who has dementia. I am challenged to bring full consciousness and unencumbered openness to whatever the person with dementia has to offer and whatever we can create together in the moment.

I invite you to dare to explore your own habitual opinions and judgments about yourself, the world and others with a light spirit and sense of play. Remember that this is not about you; it is about joining the world of the person who has dementia. To explore this shift in focus, your humor and sense of adventure will be very helpful.

HOW WE SEE OURSELVES

Several years ago, I conducted a discussion group with care professionals who perceived their past interactions with persons who have dementia as failures. They were having problems merely approaching such persons in their care. They wanted to quit or at least have all persons with dementia transferred from their case loads. I asked each care professional to come up with one word that encompassed who they were—their strongest characteristic or quality, the one they knew they could take to the bank. The following list emerged: caring, dignified, knowledgeable, loving, compassionate, intelligent, competent and classy.

I then asked them to share their examples of interactions with persons with dementia. I was not surprised that those whose most bankable qualities were "caring, loving and compassionate" thought themselves to be bad people after experiencing frustration and irritation when interacting with the person who had dementia. The people whose most valued qualities were knowledge, competence and intelligence said they felt like complete idiots when they said the totally wrong thing or found themselves tongue-tied with no idea what to say to a person with dementia. Those who named dignity and class said they felt foolish or ridiculous when they were clumsy, awkward or didn't have a clue what they were supposed to be doing. Such interactions challenged who they are—or think they are—as persons of worth.

No matter what your opinion of yourself, *OF COURSE* you will feel impatient, frustrated, stupid and foolish along the path of trying to connect with a person who has dementia. Congratulations: that means you are feeling human! It seems to be a part of our nature to be uncomfortable when entering any foreign territory, especially the very different world of the person with dementia. In no way does that mean you are a bad, or even foolish human being; you are just a human being. It is the disease that is bad and foolish because of how it damages and certainly complicates connections; the person with dementia can be in the most unpredictable places and situations from one moment to the next. Yet, the most effective focus of our effort and attention is not on the disease but on helping to make connections with the *person* inside the dementia. It is about *being with* the person. I have found that the best way to do this is to get myself and all of my opinions and judgments about myself out of the way to allow some kind of connection to unfold.

MAVIS

Mavis was 89 years old and living in an extended care facility when we met. Her dementia was quite progressed and she was on our hospice program, meaning that her physician had assessed her complicated medical condition to be so fragile that she probably had six months or less to live. The dignity, charm and sociability that she had developed during her life were fairly well intact but her language rarely made sense to those around her. She no longer recognized her children or grandchildren and most certainly didn't remember who I was from visit to visit.

During each visit with Mavis, she asked me why she was still on this earth. "God should have taken me long ago!" were the only words that she consistently stated very clearly. I encouraged Mavis to talk about her memories from different times in her life. We often looked at her family album and shared comments about all the people who were frozen in some moment from Mavis' past. Mavis had no idea who they were but her reaction to them was usually quite visceral and dramatic, often throwing out candid, partly formed phrases about their lack of fashion sense, their apparent mood, and more importantly her feelings of connection or disconnection to them. The accuracy of the details was not as important as the feelings these visual prompts evoked for Mavis. I wanted to help her search for some type of awareness of what her life has been about—to see if she could find meaning in the time she spent on earth and to discover whether she had other things to accomplish before she was to be "taken," as she phrased it.

We began each of seven weekly visits by introducing ourselves again. During each visit, Mavis wondered why she was still on earth, and during each visit we were able to superficially brush over aspects of her life with no common themes emerging. I felt there was a deeper level she was capable of reaching, yet we could not seem to get there.

My eighth visit was a little different. It began as always, except on that day, Mavis was thirsty and asked if I could get her some water. I was happy to do so. I positioned her wheel chair and locked the wheels for safety. As I stood and moved to get her cup, my spandex-blend, elastic-waistline skirt came down to my knees! Apparently, I had locked my skirt in Mavis's wheel chair. In the split second it took to reassemble myself, I searched for dignity-saving self-comforts—*Thank goodness no one else saw this. No need for embarrassment, Nancy. Easy to let this one go. As usual, all will soon be forgotten.* My thoughts were thoroughly interrupted when I looked up and saw Mavis bouncing in her chair with a fit of giggles, totally out of control. It was purely infectious and I started giggling, too. In the next moment, there we were—laughing hysterically, holding our stomachs to support our under exercised laugh muscles. People walked by and gave us looks but we did not care; we were having a pure and joyous connection in that moment.

In my preparation for our next visit I was fairly relaxed and thankful again that no one else had witnessed the skirt incident. Of course, the most forgiving aspect of Mavis' dementia was that she remembered nothing from one visit to the next—neither who I was, nor any of my unhelpful statements, fruitless explorations or fumbled attempts to relate. We could always start fresh. Many persons with dementia have helped me relax my self-judgments of ineptitude and failure by forgetting those moments about which I judged myself. Since the person let it go, I certainly could too, freeing myself for our next interaction. So—when next I walked in to visit Mavis I was not embarrassed, because the skirt incident had (virtually) NEVER HAPPENED. *Not!* Bless Mavis' wonderful heart and mind, because every time I came to visit during the next months, she said, "You're that girl whose skirt came down," and she would laugh hysterically. And so would I. From the skirt moment on, our visits were playful and joyous—healing on many levels for both of us. For me, connecting with Mavis demanded from me a deep and heart-felt surrender of my self-judgment and a willingness to develop spontaneity and the ability to laugh at myself! This was an extraordinary learning for me, further expanding my personal and professional growth.

Mavis grew too. In holding and sharing "our secret," as she once called it, Mavis opened to a deeper level of intimacy in talking about her life, dreams and hopes. As her family and I reflected back to her all that we learned from having spent time with her, Mavis came to understand that her greatest gift to the world throughout her life was, as she phrased it, "to help others fly on their own." Mavis passed away with peace and her daughter told me, with a smile on her face.

My experience with Mavis underscored for me the importance of getting myself, and my thinking about myself, out of the way so I could fully participate in the joy of our connection. Had I persisted with my opinions and judgments of stupidity, foolishness and embarrassment when my skirt came down around my knees, I would have missed the delight and intimacy we shared in that moment and in future moments.

Dare to be free of your opinions and judgments.

The Need to Know or To Be Right

I love Bill Watterson's cartoon on the next page just because it reminds me that each of us probably has more of Calvin in us than we want to admit. Calvin is that quintessential kid who lives the majority of his time in a world of his own imagination. When something shakes the reality he so dedicatedly constructed, panic sets in. The same thing happens to us. After all, we are raised being taught that our intellectual capacities are what set us apart from all other species. No wonder we fear dementia! Our society provides significant rewards for developing those capacities, for having the answers, for being *Right*. Many of us become firmly locked into our *Right* perspective of the world; other perspectives are clearly just wrong in our not-too-humble opinions. Many of us, like Calvin, become very comfortable with perspectives that provide us with a safe and orderly view of the world. To be able, even in a moment, to open to another's perspective, is to abandon what is comfortable and to enter an unrecognizable world.

If Calvin could just relax his need to *Know* or to be *Right* and live with his Dad's perspective and "unfamiliar turf" for just a few moments, he could possibly come to the understanding that he and his Dad had the potential for making a powerful connection in that moment. If he could have walked in his Dad's world and talked with him about the differences in their perspectives, they could have strengthened their bond and perhaps developed a respect for each others' points of view—neither being good nor bad, neither *Right* nor *Wrong*...just different.

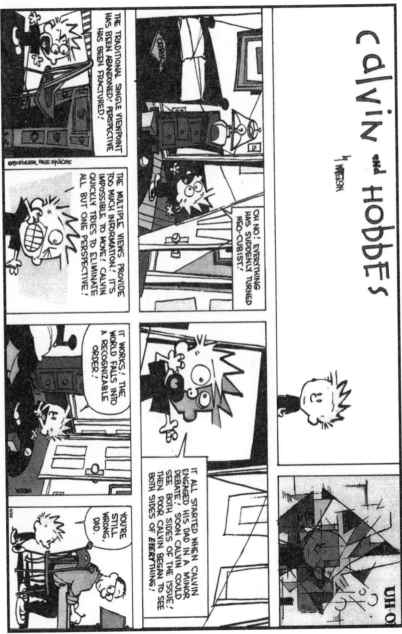

Being willing to stretch beyond your perspective is vital when connecting with persons who have dementia. By our usual standards of interacting, a person with dementia frequently communicates using words that just plain don't make sense. He reacts to things we don't see, and behaves in unpredictable ways or has moods that make it difficult for us to relate. We, of course, still remember and follow the right and appropriate traditional standards of interacting. Yet all that we know from a lifetime of traditional interactions does not serve us well when our goal is to create a connection with the person who has dementia.

Remember the example of Ida in Chapter 1? Had I remained fixated on hearing correct sentence structure and accurate wording, we would never have experienced a connection—Ida simply was not capable of giving me the words or the sentences I might have wanted to hear. Her abilities to enter my familiar world were frozen by her disease process. It was I who needed to stretch and look for ways to enter and understand Ida's world, Ida's perspective. The only way for me to connect with her was to be willing to let go of my need to hear Ida express herself in traditional ways. That mere willingness allowed me to stretch beyond my comfort zone where words and sounds have a common face value. I put aside my need to know the specifics of what was being said, and tried to listen and interact within her experience and from her perspective. The letting go and stretching is essential in creating a connection with a person who has dementia.

PEARL

Pearl was a person with dementia who rarely communicated with words but who spoke volumes in the way she gently smiled at people. She gave loving hugs to everyone she met. I would visit Pearl just to get a lift on a tough day. She always knew the gesture that would make one feel better.

On one afternoon, however, Pearl was sobbing. A dozen residents and staff immediately surrounded her trying to understand what could be the matter. We all wanted to be as helpful to Pearl as she had been to others but we were stymied about what was upsetting her. Coherent words were impossible for her; all she could do was sob. It seemed as though the more we explored, the more intense her sobbing. Perhaps Pearl was reacting much the same as we all often do—feeling insecure, embarrassed or isolated in the uncharted territory of misused words and aphasia. Perhaps Pearl was also harshly judging herself because of it.

I finally gave up looking for clues; it was clear that we weren't going to find out what was wrong by interrogating Pearl. So, I simply relaxed and focused on breathing slowly and opening myself to Pearl's experience. I realized I needed to give up my need to know what was wrong and to bring my whole focus into trying to connect with Pearl in the ways she connected with others. I looked into her tear-filled eyes and saw profound sadness. I felt guilt and frustration about not being able to figure out what had happened or how to help. Then those feelings began to fade, and a new feeling of sadness emerged—the same emotion

I thought Pearl might be experiencing. I began to be aware that I was experiencing a profound sadness that I had felt at other times in my life. My eyes also filled with tears. Pearl looked into my eyes and there it was—a very powerful connection with each other.

Pearl looked surprised, hugged me thankfully and just that quickly she was full of joy and laughter—totally transformed. It was our moment of connection that led to the transformation. The details about her sadness in that moment were really not as important to her as was the fact that someone was connecting with her. Pearl knew in those moments that she was not alone.

The compelling need to *Know*, is usually accompanied by the equally compelling need to be *Right*. Many care providers have described the dilemma they face when the person with dementia insists that his perception of the world is *Right* while the care provider *Knows* he is wrong. Years ago, those of us who were the professionals considered it helpful to orient the person with dementia to reality—that would be to *our* reality, of course. Now we have found that particularly in progressed dementia, this approach is most often ineffective and, at times, downright cruel.

MAURICE

I made a valuable discovery when watching staff orient 98-year-old Maurice to the reality that the mother he was asking for died many years ago. Each time staff told Maurice the truth, the news was brand new from Maurice's perspective. Each time he grieved deeply and was inconsolable for the rest of the day, often not even remembering why he was so upset. After each of these times, he forgot the information by the next day and asked for his mother again. It was cruel to continue to orient him to our version of reality when he was simply not able to retain the information or to process it over time.

What became very effective, however, was entering Maurice's world for the moment to get a sense of his emotion—what was behind his asking for his mother. When he was sad and missing his mother's company, we could ask questions that encouraged him to tell us about his mother and to relive some wonderful memories. Some days he was content with just our companionship, and on others he responded well when we talked about the times we missed being with our own mothers. When Maurice was worried or concerned for his mother's welfare, those of us who believed in life after death could confidently reassure him that his mother was very safe and doing well. When Maurice was upset because he needed his mother to do something for him, we let him know she could not be there at that time, but that we could certainly help him with those things. Each occasion brought a new emotion, a new exploration and a new connection with this very tender, deeply feeling man.

Only the person with dementia holds the key as to what is *Right* for him in the moment. There is no point in trying to convince the scuba diver that he should be riding in the helicopter with us (Chapter 2, page 24). It is important to ask ourselves whether specific details are all that important for the person with dementia to experience in the moment. When we relax our hold on how we see ourselves, release our need to *Know* or to be *Right* about the specifics, and dare to stretch outside our standard operating mode, we become free to explore how the person is currently experiencing his world. Being with him in his experience is how the connection will evolve.

HOW WE SEE OTHERS

PENELOPE

During my first week of my internship at the extended care facility, I met Penelope, a beautiful woman who had suffered multiple strokes that left her extremely aphasic. I clearly remember our first encounter; it was a Friday afternoon and she was very frustrated and upset. I spent a lot of time trying to understand what she was asking me. Staff and other residents stopped in to reassure me that Penelope was just confused and I should not try so hard to understand her. She kept saying something like, *ohnay habaah.* When I repeated the words, she vigorously nodded yes, thrilled that I had understood. However, I did not understand and assumed that she was misstating herself or that she was just confused as everyone had said. I tried to comfort her but seriously failed and I finally left, apologizing for not understanding her need.

One and a half hours later, I heard the overhead page announce, "Oneg Shabbat will start at 2:30." I asked staff what that meant and they told me that it was the lighting of the Sabbath candles on Friday evening. My goodness! Penelope was right on target, and I assumed she was just confused. I rushed to take her to the service. I questioned my assumptions from that point forward.

FREDA

Later that year, Freda, another resident in the same facility, provided me more insight about assumptions and how they can blur the way we see and hear persons with dementia. I was facilitating a weekly discussion group of 15 to 20 residents who shared the goal of co-writing articles for the in-house newsletter. I would record our discussion about a particular topic, transcribe it, organize the members' poignant thoughts, and then craft an article using their material. The group members were proud of their abilities to formulate thoughts, express themselves and work as a community to become published.

Freda's dementia had left her with a verbal repertoire that consisted of a monotone, "Come 'ere—Come 'ere— Come 'ere." She never expressed thoughts—didn't even seem to have any. She simply stared into space and repeated the mantra. I had never thought to bring her into a discussion group of relatively cognitively intact persons. Yet on this day, because Freda's loud repetitions could not be quieted by staff and since in the past Freda was soothed when she was seated with the other residents, the staff decided to bring her into our group.

All the regular participants became very upset, telling me that Freda should not be there, that she could not think and that she had no clue about what we were doing. Luckily, they did understand that there was no harm in her staying as long as she did not disrupt our discussion. Meanwhile, being with us had already calmed Freda and the others reluctantly allowed her to stay.

Our topic *du jour* was colors. I had brought a variety of colored sheets of construction paper and held up one color at a time to stimulate individual impressions and evoke memories. Freda sat next to me and I occasionally made eye contact and squeezed her hand to include her in the discussion, as I animated salient points. Each time, her eyes widened and eyebrows rose to reflect my expressions.

I held up the green sheet of paper and quite a few persons spoke up. Then I looked over at Freda. Her face was glowing pink, her eyes were directly focused on mine and her body was attentive and erect. I had never seen her look so alive and so beautiful. I asked what she was thinking and she said, "Green is the color of a wedding banquet in Bridgeport with flowers and greenery that were so luscious they could have been eaten." We sat dumbfounded in total silence, our mouths open in amazement. Then gradually we smiled and praised Freda for the most poetic observation of the day.

Our tendencies to assume that the person with dementia, even severe dementia, is no longer able to contribute from the richness of who she is came into question that day. The last paragraph of the article we co-created reflected the insight we experienced with Freda that day:

The world is not black and white, but is full of color. Our perceptions of each color—indeed, our perceptions of everything—are unique to each of us. How we perceive the world is not right or wrong...

it is simply unique

and colorful. (JHA ⅂⅂ , Spring, 1989)

A psychiatrist I know calls moments like the one Freda had "islands of clarity" that we witness amid a sea of confusion. These precious moments present themselves more frequently when the person who has dementia is with someone who is relaxed, open and nonjudgmentally present. They arrive more frequently when the person with dementia is treated like a *person* and not a case study, an irritant to tolerate or a disease. Dare to be free of your opinions or judgments that the person with dementia has nothing to offer or that he cannot connect.

A Note on Expectations

Those moments of experiencing a pure connection with the person who has dementia are exciting and powerful. Our desire, because we are human, is to have this level of connection with the person during each and every interaction. It is very natural to hope that such depth of connection occurs each time, but it is important to try to avoid assuming or expecting it will happen each time. To put that expectation on each visit both prevents you from being fully present with the person who has dementia and sets you up for disappointment as the person's ability to connect vacillates with the disease process. Instead, try to hold onto the feeling of those moments of connection as an inspiration and a motivation to remain open to whatever exciting new connection might be created between the two of you.

SUMMARY

The last two chapters have been about letting go of or relaxing your hold on emotional buttons and mind-sets that jam up your opportunities to create connecting interactions with persons who have dementia. When you pay attention and are willing to stretch beyond your opinions and judgments, assumptions and expectations, you will experience a new freedom in relationship to the person with dementia. When you pay attention, the person with dementia will help guide you in obvious as well as subtle ways with straight-forward feedback. He will help you come to know when you are fully present in the moment. When you pay attention, you will experience the exhilaration of being in the flow of human connectedness; you will experience the power that comes to you when you treat persons with dementia like real persons—that is, with respect, attention and nonjudgmental openness.

In the letting go, you might experience moments of feeling lost, but you also create new open space that allows the entry and evolution of moments so much more precious than you could have imagined. These moments help clarify and unite the heart and mind of both you and the person with dementia.

WORKING IT OUT

Live in the moment, release mind-sets and stretch perspectives.

Acknowledge and Celebrate Little Successes

When and if we reflect on what has gone right in our day most of us go straight to the big accomplishments and ignore—or take for granted—all the small successes that can also make us feel good. Take a few minutes right now to look back over the day for all the ways that something has gone right—including all the little ones. Here's an example of one of my daily success lists: the clerk at the Quickie Mart gave me a friendly smile this afternoon; I heard my favorite song on the radio while driving to work; I saw the first crocus in bloom; I at least got Michelle to smile a little bit; there were no complaints about what we were having for dinner tonight; that cup of coffee sure was so warm and soothing this morning; and...hey...I got up to get it! You get the idea.

Spend a few minutes every day acknowledging the seemingly insignificant things that have been right or good and start to see them as little successes. Spend a moment to appreciate and acknowledge how good those meaningful interactions, accomplishments and moments feel. Celebrate them. Committing to appreciate the small good things at the end of your day will help sustain you and transform all your days.

Expand Your Repertoire of Ways to Interact with Others

Stretch yourself beyond your everyday patterns of communication. Pay more attention to your own nonverbal communications and those of others. For example, try consciously practicing a calming physical presence, soothing vocal qualities, genuine and focused eye contact. Greet a stranger with a nod of your head, good eye contact and a gentle smile. Try experiencing your interactions through a focused act of gentle touch—when, where and with whom it is appropriate. Perhaps try breathing with the other person—matching their breathing rate. Do not do this in an obvious way, but subtly and with the intention of getting a sense as to "where the other person is" emotionally. This can help you effectively bond and/or identify with the other person.

Pay attention to what changes for you and the other during such conscious interactions.

What Would You Be?

Spend a few moments thinking about yourself. What would you say are your strongest qualities—those core essential aspects that determine who you are and how you move and interact in the world. Now ask yourself some questions that force you to think outside what you usually think about yourself:

If you were a sound, which one would you be?

If you were a piece of furniture, which one would you be?

If you were an animal, which one would you be?

If you were an automobile, which one would you be?

If you were a smell, which one would you be?

If you were a fabric, which one would you be?

"I Don't Know"

I first did this exercise in July 2001 at the Institute of Noetic Sciences Conference in California. During one of the workshops, the leaders took on what seemed to be the impossible challenge—an *I Don't Know* workout with several hundred left-brain experts. It is not an easy exercise, but many of us who ventured into it blew open our self-limiting perspectives. See if you can keep at it long enough to experience the reward of the work.

Find another person with whom you are comfortable doing an exercise. Place two chairs in position so that you can sit facing one another. Decide which one of you will ask questions first and which will answer first. You will switch roles later.

- The first person asks, one at a time, easy questions that the second person should be able to answer without having to really think. How many children do you have? What is your job? Are you married? What kind of car do you drive? What color are your eyes?

- The second person's task is not to respond in a straightforward manner. His challenge is to get himself to a place where he can very honestly respond with "I don't know." He mentally stretches to allow room for other possible meanings and interpretations of the question, until he gets to the point where he cannot answer in a brief, straightforward way.

- Nothing else is said between the two of you. The first person puts out only one question at a time and the second person responds only when he or she can honestly say "I don't know." When the response is given, the first person moves onto another simple question and the second attempts to get to unknowing again. This continues for, say, five minutes. After five minutes, switch roles and see if the first person can get to that place of, "I don't know."

Try to keep working at expanding your perspective and your traditional definitions and terminology. Explore other vantage points and amaze yourself with how you practice extending the familiar boundaries of your world. Don't worry: you can always rein it back in when you want to. In the interim, you could arrive at an awareness that enables you to solve problems or make connections that were previously beyond your reach.

4 - Love and Open to Being Loved

When I speak to care professionals about how important it is to love the person who has dementia, even in the very first moments of meeting him or her, I get a variety of reactions. Social workers and counselors are surprised—even confused—and talk to me about boundaries and professional, therapeutic distance. Others put up *no-way-am-I-going-there* resistance, and tell me it is impossible to love someone you don't even know. I tell them that not only is love appropriate and sight-unseen love possible, but it is the essential mortar in the bridge between any human being and the person with dementia. If the word *love* creates a mental block, I suggest any of the dictionary definitions: respect, honor, fondness, strong affection, admiration, tenderness, warm attachment, devotion, positive regard, compassion, mercy, gentleness, benevolence, kindness.

The Love principle works this way: when your attention, intention and focus is on loving or holding the person with dementia in tender and positive regard, you will extend real warmth into meeting him or her. This warmth of yours

creates an open, spacious and receptive likelihood for connection between you two. Without the love that you bring to
the moment, creating any kind of rapport with the person who
has dementia is a long shot.

MRS. MELIEWSKI

The social work supervisor at an extended care facility was orienting a young social work intern one afternoon
and I accompanied them. Known for her psychoanalytic
background, the supervisor possessed great knowledge
of psychological and social work theories. Her expertise,
however, had not come specifically from working with the
elderly, and it was widely known among the staff that she
still had much to learn.

Her intention that day was to model for the intern how
to greet a person who is new to the facility—how to
enter the room appropriately, help her feel welcomed
and let her know that we are always available if she needs
help adjusting to her new environment.

As we approached the room, the supervisor explained
the importance of knocking on the door and asking permission to speak with the resident. This, she said, provided choice for the person, communicated respect and
protected the resident's right to privacy and dignity. After
we entered the room correctly, the supervisor asked the
resident how she would like to be addressed. "Would you

prefer we call you Susan or Mrs. Meliewski?" The resident cautiously chose the latter. Then she added, "…at this time." It was a good beginning.

Mrs. Meliewski was a striking woman in her mid-80s. She wore a business suit, and her hair was up in a perfect twist held in place with two chop sticks. A modest amount of blush accentuated her high cheek bones. The admission paperwork stated she had mild dementia and that she had fallen several times in the previous month.

The supervisor introduced the intern and me to Mrs. Meliewski and began asking questions to discover how our new resident saw herself and how we could best support her. Mrs. Meliewski stated that she hoped her stay would be temporary and only last as long as it would take to rehabilitate, "this stupid broken hip." She shared the cursory details of her fall and then turned and looked at the supervisor. "Well you don't get to have all the questions," she said. "Where do you live?"

I have never before or since endured a more uncomfortable ten minutes of dodging a question! The supervisor's therapeutic modality asserted that giving her personal information would break the boundaries of the client-therapist relationship. "It doesn't really matter where I live," she said.

Mrs. Meliewski drew the line, "It most certainly does matter to me," she said, "and I won't answer any more of your questions until I hear an adequate response to mine."

During the standoff, Mrs. Meliewski wouldn't say a word while the supervisor struggled to appear unruffled and not irritated.

Finally, the supervisor divulged that she lived in the same town where Mrs. Meliewski had lived for 73 years but, she said, "I will not get any more specific because I just am not comfortable sharing that part of myself."

Mrs. Meliewski leaned forward and stared into her adversary's eyes, "Then, whatever-you-said-your-name-is," she said, "I'm just not comfortable sharing any of my parts, as you put it, with you."

During the next several weeks Mrs. Meliewski shared with the intern that when she turned 80 she made the choice to spend her remaining time with authentic people. "Everyone else is just a waste of time," she said, "and I do not have the time to bother with people who don't give two shakes of a lamb's tail about wanting to have a real relationship."

She didn't need to be "therapized," she said, "and I don't need people that don't know a stitch about being people around me." She said that authentic people were those whom you could trust, who weren't afraid to love and who showed respect for everyone. She asked the authentic people in her life to call her Suzie. To all the others, she remained aloof and unapproachable. She didn't have any time for what she called "those crazy games" and just wanted to "cut-to-the-chase."

Interacting with love and respect, more than any other intention, creates authentic interactions with the person who has dementia. It is basic cutting-to-the-chase, as Mrs. Meliewski so aptly put it. It is a state of being that enables me to bring honesty, warmth and respect into whatever direction our time together takes. By focusing on love and centering myself in the open-hearted spacious feeling that accompanies it, I take responsibility for beginning the bridge to connection. And because the person with dementia can easily read my face, body posture and voice, a bridge to connection is much more probable if I am in a loving place than if I am in some other condition—such as, mentally rehashing an argument from earlier in the day.

The important question remains, however, how can I love a person who has dementia when I don't know or have just met her? First of all, in reality none of us knows the person with dementia in any moment. She might be unfamiliar to even family and lifelong friends because of the shifting of the disease process. There is no way to predict her reactions or her potential abilities to interact. As we knock on her door, we truly do not know her, whether or not we are meeting for the very first time.

So, how do we center ourselves in love and extend that love into the forever-new interaction with the person who has dementia? There are several ways into our own heart territory. One is to remember the nature of the disease and its impact on the person with dementia.

ACCESSING LOVE THROUGH UNDERSTANDING

One of my teachers, Frédéric Lionel, often said, "Understand so as to love." If I understand that the disease process interferes with the individual's ability to interact and behave in familiar ways, then I will be more open to loving the person inside the disease. If I understand that it is the destroyed brain tissue that causes the person's problem behaviors and not her lack of control or willpower, I will most likely be less reactive and more compassionate. If I understand that structural changes in the brain can change emotions, personality and ability to reason, then I can see beyond those manifestations of the disease and instead choose to respect the strengths and challenges of the person.

I have seen how just a little understanding of the disease can empower family and care providers with love and resiliency. It made a difference to Claire to understand that her uncle did not urinate in her flowers because he had suddenly stopped liking her, developed control issues or was out for revenge. It was important for Bob to know that his mom did not pack and unpack her suitcase all night long just to drive him crazy from sleep deprivation. It helped Yolanda to know that Paulette did not dress with her bra on top of her blouse so she could get attention and make more work for staff. Each of these care providers had been spinning between hurt and rage, exhaustion and restless anxiety—because of the disease process, not because of the person with the disease.

When these care persons understood and accepted that it was the disease and not the person with the disease that had them in reactive nose-dives, something changed for the better. They became less concentrated on the behaviors and more open to discovering ways to interact with and be responsive to the person with dementia. This made them able then to access love for the person with dementia.

ACCESSING LOVE THROUGH WHAT'S LOVEABLE

When I discover something I truly admire or like about the person with dementia, I get a key into my own state of loving. I can think about that aspect and let it fill my heart with admiration as I enter the room and greet her. When my heart is warm and positive, I greet her without agenda, prejudice, or anticipation—I am very simply opening to interact with whatever aspect of her that makes me feel positive. Here are a few avenues for discovering those aspects that will help bring you into loving exchanges with the person who has dementia.

The Common Bond

DANIEL

Daniel was a devoted son who had a difficult time in his mother's decline. Suzanne, his mother, was nearing the end of an eleven-year journey with Alzheimer's disease. Daniel and his wife had cared for Suzanne in their home for eight years, and when they could no longer physically handle her care, they placed her in a skilled nursing facility. Daniel was actively involved with his mother's care team and spent a lot of time either educating himself about the disease or being by his mother's side as her abilities to interact with the world changed. In her current debilitated state, however, Daniel had a very hard time going to visit his mother. She was bed-ridden; her arms and legs were contracted, her sky-blue eyes never focused on him anymore. Each time he visited, he could only see the ravages of the disease and not his mother. Understanding how the disease process created the changes in his mother had helped him remain connected to her through eleven years. Now, however, he struggled to find what, here and now, he could relate to with love.

Daniel and I were sitting one afternoon in the family room on his mother's unit as he told me what was going on for him. Heavy snow was coming down outside and as Daniel watched the storm through the window, he shared memories of snow play when he was a boy. He would stay outside until he was just shy of frost bite, having every last minute of fun he could. When he finally did come inside, his mother would meet him with clean dry clothes that she had warmed on the radiator. "That's who my mother has always been," he said, "a woman who showed us her love through the little things like those toasty warm clothes after I played in the snow. We knew with every gesture that she loved us."

Daniel heard his own words and realized that he resolved his issue. From that moment on, he was able to go into his mother's room with his heart full of love. All he did was remember any one of the little things his mother did to show her love over the years and he walked in with that feeling of having just been hugged by her. His mother was no longer hidden by the disease. "I began to see the color return to her face as I sat with her," he said. "Her body became less tense when I held her hand and rubbed her arms. And, I swear, that she turned the corner of her mouth up for a smile every now and then. My mother taught me that the little things really do matter. I discovered that being there with love in little ways was powerful for both of us."

Family members and friends often find the focus on common bonds shared across time to be very helpful in remaining connected to their loved one. These long-term relationships have a rich dimensionality and depth that cannot be matched by someone just now entering the life of the person with dementia. The challenge, however, is often in having to deal with the feelings associated with losing the person they once knew or the unresolved conflicts which resurface. When the balance can be found, as it did with Daniel, the ensuing connection is profound.

Interestingly enough, the common-bond approach can be helpful even if you have no history at all with the person. If you can, find out a little about the person with dementia before your interaction with her. This gives you a chance to see if you can relate positively to any of her qualities or aspects of her history. Perhaps you can respect *her* passion for needlepoint because you can't relax at the end of your day without spending time on your own needlepoint. Perhaps you like the fact that she has a favorite cousin who lives in Wisconsin, because you do too. Perhaps she owned a beauty shop just like your aunt, whom you dearly loved.

Finding some common bond can bring on very warm feelings that put you in an open loving state as you cross the threshold into initial moments with the person who has dementia.

A Personality Trait

Perhaps the person's personality or way of interacting reminds you of someone in your own life whom you love or loved once upon a time. Some personalities certainly seem to be easier to love than others, but it is possible that even the most ostensibly difficult persons can still have an attraction. For example, I *LOVE* working with the person who barks orders, or throws staff out of the room or complains endlessly—the person at the crusty-cranky end of the personality spectrum. I thoroughly respect the strength of her convictions, and the fight for dignity as she experiences the effects of her disease.

This wasn't always the case. I started with my connection with Doris, the avid complainer with a hidden sense of humor (Chapter 2, page 28). Interacting with the type-Gruff personality warms my heart with memories of the challenges I faced and the transformation Doris experienced. During that first year of my internship, I learned the great value of being patient enough to allow my relationship with Doris to take shape one thin layer of connection at a time. When I focus on this memory of my experience with Doris, I am less reactive to how the disease presents itself and more open to discovering details about the person that don't at first meet the eye. As a result, I enter that initial interaction with enthusiasm about meeting the person inside the barking persona.

I know it is just a matter of time before we connect and I look forward to seeing how it will play out. I am not defended; I am excited. I don't have a fearful or intimidated look on my face because I am thinking about my positive experiences with other cranky persons in the past. I don't fold my arms for self-protection or put my hands on my hips—the universal sign of irritation. My whole body is relaxed and open to whatever will happen in the moment. Relaxed body language alone, in fact, can greatly increase opportunities for connecting with the person who has dementia. She is not stupid. She picks up all the signals and most often responds authentically to whatever is coming her way.

Strengths

I have been greatly influenced by the work of Carel Germain and Alex Gitterman (*The Life Model of Social Work Practice*), Agnes Hatfield (*Families of the Mentally Ill: Coping and Adaptation*) and Lois Murphy and Alice Moriarty (*Vulnerability, coping, and growth*). In defining the therapeutic relationship, these authors focus on the client's strengths and abilities, rather than seeing a constellation of pathologies to be weeded through and eliminated. This perspective asks us to look at the person herself rather than her disease or dysfunction. We are interested therefore in her potential to adapt to her current situation and we boost any environmental supports that can help her express that potential.

Sometimes a person's strengths jump right out and you readily relate. It might be Bill's sense of humor for example, or Sophia's ability to express her feelings, even when her words are disjointed. Christina might be able to mobilize resources, and you admire how she uses support to maximize her independence and self-sufficiency. You may be drawn to Gordon's powerful sense of hope and faith, and even take comfort when you hear him say, "With God's help, we'll get through this whole thing with grace."

CHANGE THE FRAME

Sometimes a person's strengths do not jump right out, however, and in order to see them you need a new frame, a new way of seeing and thinking about the person.

When my grandmother moved from her two-story home into a smaller place she gave away many possessions. There was one drawing that I thought stunning—a winter-night scene done mostly in dark-blue pastels. The matting and frame were so ugly that no one wanted it, so it easily became mine.

Eventually, I changed the matting and the frame. Family and friends who had seen the picture over the years could not believe mine was the same one. Because the new framing brought out the art work's strengths and beauty, people had entirely new reactions to and appreciation of the work.

The principle of reframing works in all relationships and especially with persons who have dementia. Strengths and other character qualities can easily be seen when we decide to look at the person with a slightly different frame or perspective. Here are a few examples:

GARY

Gary's dementia turned him into "the most stubborn of men" according to his son. Everything had to go his way, in his time frame and be delivered to him—with a smile. As the staff at the skilled facility got to know him over time, we began to appreciate the underpinnings of his stubbornness. Gary certainly had the greatest capacity for the struggle that we had ever seen. He loved challenges and he introduced us to playfulness in banter. He taught us about his life lessons—the strength to be found in assertiveness and commitment to determination.

MRS. WILLIAMS

Mrs. Williams could no longer talk or waltz; she had won state championships in ballroom dancing twelve times during the 1930s and 1940s. "Dancing had been her life," her daughter said. "What a loss for her not to be able to even stand now." However, whenever we would bring her into a group with music, and we could see her still dancing with her eyes, her shoulders, her spirit. Mrs. Williams still had a great capacity for enjoyment and for relating to others through dance; it was simply dance in a different form. Her daughter grew to love her mother's new way of dancing as her way of staying connected with her mother.

MONA

Mona regularly became upset in the late afternoons as the sun went down—the behavior pattern called sundowning affects many persons with dementia. She could feel the discomfort mounting but could not verbalize why she was upset. Since the onset of her dementia, however, she had been able to identify what helped her during those difficult times—her stuffed animal, a Golden Labrador Retriever. So, as she began to get upset, Mona reached for her Lab, hugged it and broadly smiled as she rocked backward and forward. Her family was upset with this behavior. "She looks and acts like a child," they said. "Where's the dignity in that!?" Yet when they began to see that Mona had an extraordinary capacity for self-healing and self-comforting they honored her way of coping and opened to her with love.

HILDA

Hilda, Nan's mother, spoke in barbs to keep people away. "What happened to my mother?" Nan wanted to know. "She's turned into such a grumpy old biddy. She used to be the most sociable person around." Hilda sat outside her room and knit, refusing to get involved in what she called "nonsensical, fluff conversations." "The work is too important," she said.

We discovered that Hilda was on a knitting mission that began just after her diagnosis of Alzheimer's Disease. She was making afghans, lap throws and sweaters for the elderly and homeless. Hilda's ability to receive gratification from her work, her satisfaction in her accomplishments, her commitment to a higher cause and her generosity to the extended community began to shine through over time. This new frame helped bring understanding and acceptance from those around her.

As Joanne Koenig Coste, author of *Learning to Speak Alzheimer's,* reminds us, "Don't ever spend so much time looking at who they used to be that you miss the very special person they are." The beauty and the strengths are there—perhaps framed in a different way from in the past, but they most certainly are there. The person's strengths are the adaptations she makes to the changes that occur in each moment. Her strengths lie in everything that creates that personal spark in her life. When you discover those strengths and relate to the person with dementia through them, you have a powerful avenue for connection. You are also dramatically supporting the expression of his and her potential.

If that strength is one that you personally relate to or identify with, then bring the positive feeling it engenders into the initial moment with the person who has dementia and watch the connection between you unfold.

Use Your Senses

At times, your senses will be the pathway to discovering what you like or admire about the person with dementia and will encourage a loving interaction.

SIGHT

Some of us take in information primarily in a visual way. Think of a favorite person or place, and if an image rather than a string of words comes to mind, you are probably in this visual category. To experiment further, imagine the person or place and close your eyes. If the image becomes very clear and so do your feelings for that person or place, then it is possible that your inroad to what is "loveable" in the person with dementia is going to be a visual one. Here are a few examples of what I mean.

VERNA

Verna lived in a skilled facility and was bedridden due to the severe progression of her disease. The first time I entered Verna's room, the shades were pulled, the lights were off and I could barely see a thing. I introduced myself briefly and asked if it was OK to open the curtains to let in a little light. She did not respond. The staff had told me she hadn't said a word in over a year. I went over to open the curtains and noticed that Verna's eyes followed me. When the light came into the room, I looked over at Verna and saw her exquisite long white hair flowing in curls and providing the perfect frame for her flawless, porcelain complexion. How could it be that this woman has lived for 89 years and has such perfect skin, I thought! There I was at age 53, with far more signs of wear-and-tear than Verna. I was in awe. As I more fully introduced myself to Verna, I told her what I had just been seeing and thinking. She grinned and said very tenderly, "Oh, thank you."

BEATRICE

Beatrice reached out to greet me on the first day we met, with hands that were extremely bent and twisted from years of hard work—and arthritis, I assumed. She was apologetic, but I was in awe of the sight. Her hands immediately reminded me of my favorite Aunt Kally, whose hands, like those of Beatrice, were a map of her life. Aunt Kally had been my strong female role model as I was growing up; she always made me feel loved and worthy. Seeing Beatrice's hands brought me back to the strong loving connections with my aunt. These warm, loving feelings were present that first day and in all my subsequent interactions with Beatrice. What a great jumping-off place for connection.

KAREN

Karen's environment provided me with a visual road to connection. She was a woman who loved rainbows. Her daughters were committed to honoring Karen's wish to remain in her home for her final months. When the time came to get a hospital bed, they set it up in the front room—a room with a big picture window overlooking the stream and the forest. It was Karen's favorite room because the sun streamed through that window during the afternoons and a dozen different crystals cast rainbows all about the room. Each afternoon, Karen delighted in the dancing colors around and within her. Through that visual, she shared her dance with me. What a gift!

SOUND

MR. GILLMORE

Mr. Gillmore exuded contentment with life even though he had lost just about everything: his vision was gone due to macular degeneration, he could not hear even with the help of devices and his physical and cognitive abilities had been ravaged by disease and dementia. And yet, as I approached him for the first time, I heard a deep and slow sound, a hummmmmm as he exhaled on each breath. The sound was soothing and content as was the look on his face. When he became aware of my presence, he showered me with God-bless-you's and thank-you's. As years passed and Mr. Gillmore was no longer able to hum or speak, my strong memory of his contented sounds and grateful words filled me with love and joy as I approached each new connection with him.

FREDA

Remember Freda who repetitively said, "Come 'ere—Come 'ere—Come 'ere," in a pounding monotone (Chapter 3, page 61)? There was no urgency in her relentless chant, and even after much exploration on our part, we could rarely find an apparent need that warranted our attention. No matter how we tried to "Come 'ere" for Freda, the non-stop verbalizations continued. Her daughter told us that Freda had been "a talker her whole life, whether or not anyone was there to listen." She supposed it was "kind of a self stimulation." The incessant chanting, however, became quite irritating to everyone. Residents and staff alike often either ran away or tried to distract Freda long enough to get a break from the constant repetition. Then the day came when Freda was no longer able to speak and it surprised us all how we missed her "Come-'ere, Come-'ere." For staff and residents alike, Freda's chant had become a significant part of our daily ambient sound—the sound that brought consistency and calm to our otherwise unpredictable and crazy days. We warmly and lovingly thought of those sounds as we cared for her during her declining months.

According to a study published in the *Journal of Geronto-logical Nursing*, when baroque music was played during meal-time at a long term care facility, the verbally and physically agitated behaviors of persons with Alzheimer's disease decreased by more than 55 percent. It's no wonder. Music and rhythms connect people to their past, to each other and to their souls. In my experience, music can open every heart in the room, which is the quintessential green light for authentic interaction and connection. I resonated right away with Paul's love of Frank Sinatra, whose singing filled the house while Paul reminisced about playing trumpet in Sinatra's band. Marjorie and I would jump and jive with joy during our visits because of her love of big band music. Sadie reverberated in spirit and soul as we shared singing and listening to gospel music. The keys for us are to find and share the music that can give the person pleasure and understand that her preferences might shift depending on the activity or the time of day.

SMELL AND TASTE

AUNTIE Z

I used to love to go to Auntie Z's home. She had no children of her own, yet according to her nieces she was the best mother anyone could have. All three nieces set up a schedule so that one of them was always with Auntie Z during the day; a professional care person stayed during the nights. Thursdays were my days to visit and they were also apple pie days. Even though my friend, Elizabeth, was an accomplished baker, on Thursdays she asked and allowed her Auntie Z to teach her how to make a pie. From Auntie Z's perspective, each lesson was Elizabeth's first. By the time I stepped over the threshold, the pie was cooling and the wafting smell of cinnamon would bring me right back to memories of my grandmother's pies and her cinnamon cookies. How could I not enter the presence of Auntie Z and Elizabeth with love? When it was time to taste test their baking, it was my role to be the objective stranger—a tough job but someone has to do it, right? When I smacked my approval, the accolades always brightened Auntie Z—or, as Elizabeth said, "they lifted her soul."

JULIE

Carrie, a home-care nurse, told me how the smell of honeysuckle changed her interactions with Julie, who at 73 was in early dementia. Carrie visited often to tend to Julie's leg sores and change the dressings. Carrie described going to Julie's house as oppressive—the shades were always drawn and the air was stale and dank; the windows had been probably locked for years. Carrie was tense and irritated in the house. Her interactions were not very fulfilling either—Julie was always timid and quiet. One day, on her way up the walk to Julie's house, Carrie smelled the honeysuckle which lined the path. "That fragrance brought me back to the home where I raised my children," she told me, "I loved that time in my life so much."

When Carrie entered the house that day, everything changed. She enjoyed being there and Julie was sociable, smiling and energetic. As she left, Julie invited her back saying, "You were so much nicer today than the other times." Carrie realized in that moment that it was she who was different that day. Instead of entering the house tense and irritated as in the past, she entered with open hearted and loving memories that the smell of the honeysuckle had elicited. Carrie reflected, "I learned on that day how my open heart can transform my experience of nearly anything."

JANET

Janet's use of lavender was overpowering. I have never been a fan of perfume and lavender in particular is usually splashed, sprayed or dabbed on too lavishly for me. And even though Janet might have lost her sense of smell and her judgment about how much perfume was too much, she did not lose her joyous impulse to give any one of us, at any time, one of her great big bear hugs. The good news is that I thoroughly loved those hugs! It didn't take long to put together the smell of lavender with Janet being just yards away, and I was about to get one of the world's greatest hugs. Now, the scent of lavender carries a positive memory for me and sometimes I use the scent to remind me of Janet; it opens my heart to whatever comes next.

TOUCH

MRS. GILBERT

Mrs. Gilbert was at the point in her long decline where she was not actively interacting with others but spending her days in a hospital bed. So, her children decided that the best they could do for her was to surround her with softness. They would try, they said, "to make her world a heaven on earth, to make her feel like she was floating on a cloud." Everything in her room was soft—the floating mattress, 1000 thread count Egyptian cotton bed linens and nightgowns, gentle warmth of the indirect sunlight through the windows and body lotions. Absolutely everything in her room was exquisite to touch, particularly Mrs. Gilbert's hands. Spending time with her was calming for me. Holding her hand made me feel nurtured even as I was nurturing.

BETTY

Betty's gift to the world was in her touch. I first met her one afternoon on the dementia care unit where she had been living for five months. As the afternoon progressed and the busy sounds intensified on the unit, Betty set herself and her wheel chair into motion. She rolled from room to room and very calmly held each person's hand, gently patted their forearm and lightly hugged their shoulder. There were no words or conversation, just her touch. Even our grouchiest resident, Mr. Garner, allowed Betty to shake his hand. Her touch transformed the people around her—I could see it in their faces and in the way their bodies relaxed in her presence.

HILDA

Hilda had survived World War II *and* Auschwitz and she had been a housekeeper at one skilled care facility for 37 years when I met her. At 82, she had no intention of ever retiring. Hilda poured love into her work and her interactions with residents on the units. She told me that she loved being with the confused persons through her touch. "It's in the hands, you know," she said. "All you have to do is hold the person's hand and you'll just get it. You'll get it that this is a human being, a creature of God…just like yourself. How can you not open to the love?"

THE HEALING POTENTIAL OF OPENING TO LOVE

As I hope you can see, there are many ways to look for—and find—the thing about another person that will open you to feeling love, tenderness or respect for her. Choosing to do this puts you at ease and, almost automatically, lets your heart flow into a loving interaction. Focus totally on that unique aspect; fully celebrate and admire it—his strength, her spark, his emotional openness, her manners that remind you of your grandmother, his struggle for dignity revealed by his insisting on wearing a tie every day. You will fill up with positive emotions of admiration, inspiration even delight. As you practice focusing on what is loveable before as many interactions as possible with the person with dementia, at the very least you will bring respect, tenderness and compassion as you acknowledge each person's ability to do the best she can under the barrage of the disease process. This practice takes just a few moments of your attention, and it has the power to form and transform the moments you spend with each person.

As you approach the person with dementia while thinking about what you like and admire about her, you enter the moment in an open and positive state. She sees and hears this in your body stance, your voice, your facial expressions and your words— possibly without you even being aware of your physical and vocal qualities. You become calm and as gently relaxed as a close friend because you are holding in your heart the positive feelings that you associate with the person who has dementia. All these manifestations of the shift you have made toward loving are known to be effective in interacting with persons who have dementia. Yet it appears that the impact of our loving presence is far beyond these things we can immediately identify.

Exciting research is being done at the Institute of HeartMath in Boulder Creek, California, the results from which are published in *The HeartMath Solution* and *Transforming Stress: The HeartMath Solution for Relieving Worry, Fatigue, and Tension*. Their research shows that positive emotions such as compassion, caring, love and joy produce smooth or more ordered heart rhythm patterns. These smooth rhythms correlate to lowering blood pressure, the release of stress-reducing hormones, increased immune responses and brain function that supports clear and efficient thinking. We just plain feel better physically, mentally and emotionally. More jagged or disordered heart rhythm patterns on the other hand result from stressful emotions, and tend to correlate to the opposite of all the good things produced by positive emotions.

Even more pertinent to my work, some of the research shows how heart rhythms, both smooth and irregular, produce electromagnetic signals that impact others. The heart's electrical field has been measured to extend beyond the body up to ten feet. This is only as far as equipment can measure at this time! Just as important, the electromagnetic signals that emit from the rhythms of a person's heart have also been measured in the brain waves of other persons around her. This study indicates that we are literally making waves as we feel our emotions and those waves affect the heart rhythms and brain waves of the persons around us. This *energetic nonverbal communication* via heart rhythms *produces an immediate and deep understanding and connection between human beings.*

So, when we enter each moment with positive emotions and their associated smooth heart rhythms, we help the person with dementia to do the same. Smooth heart rhythms give each of us a greater potential for adapting to stressful events, for improving overall health and well-being and for improving communications—we are maximizing our potential for connection. The connections may be very subtle and may be beneath our levels of awareness, but they are real. Both of us feel the benefits. Being on the same positive wave, then, is a potent "win-win" situation.

These research results are not a surprise to any one of us who has seen how persons with dementia easily connect to the person who is openhearted and loving. At times, the person with dementia far exceeds our expectations of her ability to not only make a connection but also to express love. And when that happens, it illumines an all-important aspect of our work: being open to receiving the love that comes back at us.

OPEN TO BEING LOVED

Let's say that you have successfully discovered something associated with the person who has dementia that you honestly respect, admire or love and you have let your heart fill with these emotions when you are with the person. You have seen the positive effect of your loving state of being on the person with dementia and, most likely, this has made you feel wonderful.

It's a great start, but only a start. Our aim here is *connecting with* the person with dementia, not simply giving her love. It is about the give-and-take rhythm of humans being connected—not about unilaterally spreading good vibes.

When you fill your heart with loving compassion and intention, the person with dementia will resonate on more levels than probably any of us can quantify. And turnabout is fair play—and natural! When you allow the person with dementia to demonstrate that she can have a positive impact on someone else...YOU, then you have an opportunity to bring her back into the kind of human connection that, due to the ravages of the disease process, becomes beyond reach for so many. To do so, it is important that you remain open to her expressions of affection that will be returned to you. It is important to be open to *being loved*.

I know that it is difficult for many of us to receive love. We are so much more capable of giving than taking it in. One of the most revealing exercises for me over the years was during my social work training. Each of us was paired off with another student. Our direction was to take turns verbally expressing appreciations to each other (see third *Working It Out* at end of this chapter). The task of the person receiving the appreciation was to accept it without debate or denial. In the discussion after the exercise it was unanimous—we all had no problem whatsoever giving appreciations, but had all kinds of difficulty receiving them. It was a major struggle to keep our internal and verbalized disclaimers silent—let alone to accept what was being said. Most of us had difficulty opening fully enough to allow the appreciations to touch our hearts. However, doing just that, letting in another person's appreciation and affection, is key to completing your give-and-take connection with the person who has dementia.

When you receive love that manifests from the person with dementia, you are open to being affected and changed by that person just as she is being affected and changed by you. When you allow her to touch your heart, she sees that she has influenced you in a positive way and she feels good. She moves out of her isolation and both of you enter what Drs. Miller and Stiver in *The Healing Connection* call an *authentic, mutually enhancing relationship*. Each of you gains a sense of well-being by being in touch with the other and acting on positive thoughts and feelings.

At times, the person with dementia will express love very directly. Such was my experience with Ida, the woman I mentioned in the first chapter who said, "I love you. You treat me like such a person." When that happened, I was stunned. For almost two years, Ida had been unable to effectively verbalize anything—but there she was, very clearly and warmly expressing her love. She had no capacity to play games, no ability or memory of intentions to manipulate, no ulterior motives. Her expression of love was authentic; her words came straight from her heart and into mine. I was touched deeply and when Ida noticed my reaction, a very contented look of pleasure came over her face.

She knew she had returned my love with an extraordinary gift of her own and that moment of reciprocity made her feel wonderful, too. Within a very short time, the moment of clarity passed and she continued on as before. That experience of expressed love and appreciation, however, deepened our connection from that day forward.

At times, the person's love comes to you in unique and creative ways. Remember Gary, "the most stubborn of men" (Chapter 4, page 80)? On Gary's first day at the facility, frantic staff paged me to step in when he went into a rage and began throwing furniture around his room. At 78, Gary's dementia had progressed to the point where he could no longer live safely in his home of 53 years. Gary's son, the court-appointed conservator, decided to move him to the extended-care facility. Gary was furious. "They are the crazy ones, not me," he yelled as I dodged a flying chair. "I am the only sane one in the bunch!" I'll talk more in detail in the next chapter about what can be helpful in transforming this type of anger. For the point of this example, we were able to help Gary calm himself that day. He had spent his adult life as an accomplished sculptor and we eventually assisted him in finding constructive outlets for his extraordinary creative energies.

Five months after our first encounter, Gary came to my office and placed on my desk a little chair that he had meticulously carved out of a block of sponge. He said with his signature grumpy style, "I suppose it's fair that you get to throw a chair back at me." I laughed and accepted this gift from his heart. When he saw my delight, the circle was complete—he knew I heard the apology, saw the humor and accepted the loving gesture. That was the day we first saw Gary smile. And what a great smile it was! His gruff personality made a shift that day, and from then on we saw Gary smile a lot.

Sometimes the simplest gestures express love from the person with dementia: Karen reached for my hand the moment she noticed that I also took great joy in the rainbows dancing about her room. That was an extraordinary moment for me—it brought tears to our eyes and a long, focused gaze of silent communication.

Betsy tenderly moved a lock of my hair from my eyes; Mrs. Williams winked and smiled after enjoying a dance; Mrs. Gilbert took a deep breath and made a comforting sigh when I held her hand. I was changed by these expressions of appreciation and love and felt even more loving toward each person.

Each person's impact on me was noticeable, being expressed in my face, my demeanor or nonverbally, through the energetic communications in the shifting of my heart rhythms. Yet the impact was clear...my heart was touched by each. We were on the same playing field—each of us open to being touched by the other, to expressing (one way or another) our thoughts or feelings about having been touched. Our connection came full circle and was mutually beneficial and empowering. We experienced the healing connection that Drs. Miller and Stiver describe in their book by that name.

Drs. Miller and Stiver describe how a healing connection deepens each person's sense of well-being through their being in touch with the other. We find ways to act on our thoughts and feelings and see that our actions are understood and received by the other. These bonds increase each person's pleasure, sense of worth, effectiveness and vitality.

SUMMARY

During the time you spend with the person who has dementia, you will have extraordinary opportunities to explore ways each of you can participate in the rhythm of human connectedness. By bringing a loving intention into your moments together, you begin to bridge the chasm between you. You take responsibility for the first step. The effect of the principle of **Love and Open to Being Loved** is the enrichment of each person. It becomes a growth cycle.

Interacting with the intention of love in your heart while you are open to receive love creates moments of rapport without the usual social or psychological games. It allows you to communicate beyond words that you honor and respect the person with dementia however she reveals herself to you. These interactions hold the potential for powerful transformations for both of you.

What if we can't really feel those connections with the person who has dementia? What if we aren't sure that "magic" is happening? Is there something else we "should" be doing? Is there something else that could be helpful? First of all, we need to not panic! We need to just relax and let go of our gremlins, remember? We need to be patient with a process that might take some time to unfold. It is fair, however, to wonder what else we can do to help create connection with the person who has dementia.

WORKING IT OUT

Love and open to being loved.

Discover the Little Things that Open the Heart

Do you know someone who never gets ruffled even in times of crisis? I have met a few and have asked for the secret to their balance and calming presence:

- A nurse I knew knocked or tapped the same five rhythmic beats whenever she entered someone's room or a crisis situation. She said it was the rhythm at the beginning of a lullaby sung to her throughout her childhood. She said this tapping reminded her to enter each moment with pure love and caring.
- Several people hum a soothing song. Sometimes, the song is associated with a comforting memory; other times, it is the vibration in the chest that loosens tensions.
- Some people focus on a favorite piece of jewelry—a ring or necklace given to them by a beloved grandmother, for example. Touching or looking at such heirlooms helps some reconnect with caring, respectful, loving feelings in the moments about to be entered.
- Three people told me they carry a little rock or crystal discretely in their pocket. Touching it helps remind them of their connection with the *Earth Mother* or with the grounding energy of the universe.

- Sometimes, people carry a rosary or a Tibetan mala (beads) with them to continually remind them of their loving connection with God. One young Jewish woman used to touch the mezuzah she imagined on the frame of each doorway she approached to remind her of God's words.

- Smelling a touch of perfume, flower essence or anointing balm dabbed on the inside of the wrist has been helpful for many people in aiding relaxation and an open heart.

- Several people read from a small, easily accessible laminated card containing a favorite poem, biblical reference or sayings that inspire compassion, kindness and gentleness in the moment. A few healthcare professionals told me they hang a laminated card showing the **IF LOST** concepts from their identification holder as a reminder before interactions, particularly with a person who has dementia. [See the end of this book for a business-card-sized cutout containing a brief summary of the concepts.]

Take a few minutes right now to think about some of your own private ways to rekindle and connect with good feelings and love. These very simple reminders can be powerful tools of support in every situation.

Open the Heart to Love

A quiet moment or two of conscious breathing and focused meditative images can loosen defenses and open your heart to love. Judith Blahnik, my dear friend, wrote the following exercise and uses it during her presentations and workshops to encourage adults and children to open their hearts.

Sit comfortably with your hands in your lap and close your eyes. Take a few breaths to relax your shoulders, arms and chest muscles; each time you breathe in, imagine sending your breath into your shoulders, then into your arms, then into your chest. Allow the breath to flow into and through those muscles until they are relaxed.

Now think about your heart, and listen. Place your hand on the center of your chest; be very still and just listen to your heart. If you begin to think about other things, gently bring your focus back to your heart.

Now expand your focus to include your breathing. With each slow inhalation, imagine sending your breath into your heart. With each exhalation imagine your breath flowing through and out of your heart. Find a rhythm that is comfortable for you. (I inhale for 8 counts and exhale for 8 counts). Do this several times until the image of your breath flowing into and out of your heart comes easily and smoothly.

As you continue this breathing, expand your focus once again to include images of persons, places or things that evoke feelings of love, appreciation and caring. As the image becomes clear and the positive feelings rise up within you, let the image and the feelings ride the breath into and through your heart. As your heart fills with breath, so does it fill with feelings of love, appreciation and caring. Do this several times, or until you have found a comfortable rhythm.

This entire exercise can take one minute or as long as you want it to take. No matter how much time you spend, the result is the same. It opens your heart to all the positive feelings that already belong to you, that are always yours to have and to share.

Open the Heart to Being Loved

Find another person with whom you feel comfortable doing an exercise. Place two chairs facing each other, and sit down. Decide which of you will speak and which will listen first. You will switch roles later.

The speaker describes in words some positive qualities that she authentically appreciates about the other, taking time to fully express that those qualities have made an impression on her or have touched her heart.

The listener's task is to receive the appreciation and to simply take it in—that's right, no verbal or nonverbal debates, denials or disclaimers. This includes no snickers or smirks, no looks like you know this first person is crazy, no "harrumphs" and no looking away. Your only task as the listener task is to turn off the brain's tendency to come up with disclaimers, and fully breathe the affirmations in and through your heart—feel what it is like to fully take them in.

Now switch roles.

5 - Silence and the Art of Being With the Person who has Dementia

FRAN

Fran was not the most subtle communicator as her dementia progressed. Whenever anyone tried to engage her in a dialogue, she frowned, rocked in her chair, shook her head and said, "TALK-talk-talk-talk-talk-talk, TALK-talk-talk-talk-talk-talk." Perhaps she was unable to process our words or was irritated that she couldn't gather her own. Or maybe we were intruding on her private thoughts: even as word usage diminishes, the person with dementia still has thoughts and experiences. Whatever her reasons, Fran's message was clear: she wanted less talk and more silence during our interactions with her.

Silence, however, was uncomfortable for many members of the care team. Most of us were not used to connecting with others in silence, and our little gremlins filled any quiet airspace with inner negative chatter in a split second (see Chapter 2). We were on rough turf when we had no words to pave the way; and those gremlins were quick to point out our deepest insecurities, fears, impatience, grief and inadequacies. We became easily distracted, making it impossible to be fully present in the moment.

Even if we could give our gremlins some time off and focus an intention to connect with Fran, we often got trapped in our assumptions and opinions about the down-side of Fran's silence (see Chapter 3). Some of us had compelling beliefs about her need to speak— "use it or lose it." Others believed that there was no potential for real connection with Fran without some verbal exchange. Some team members easily slid into assuming what Fran wanted and quickly jumped into problem-solving before fully considering the silence from Fran's perspective. Most had no difficulty keeping lips zipped and maintaining outward silence with Fran. The most significant challenge, particularly during extended periods of silence, was keeping our *minds* quiet.

When the wisdom and spiritual traditions teach about silence, they rarely mean the mere surrendering of words—outer silence. Frédéric Lionel would say, "Be silent when words are superfluous." This teaching challenges me to go beyond the holding of my tongue to stilling my mind. There are a variety of terms for this kind of silence: inner stillness, quiet mind, peace, self control, calming of the mind, surrendering words and tranquility of the soul.

Deep inner silence is constantly challenged during our interactions with a person who has dementia, and yet, in my experience it is essential. When I focus on calming my mind, I open more readily and fully to communicating through the heart. My heart rhythms become smooth and my nonverbal communications with others transcend the barriers created by the illness (Chapter 4, page 94). Only in such inner silence can I put aside my perception of my world, enter the world of the person with dementia and fully 'listen' to what he is communicating in the moment. This listening in silence is not passivity; it is whole, attentive presence.

ZELDA

I met Zelda when I was a very green social work student. In her late 90's then, Zelda had been at the facility for seven years and was initially admitted because of a "failure to thrive" out in the community. Little was known of her history—her family and friends had long since died and no one could validate her own verbal reports. As I walked into her unit that first day, Zelda was sitting near the nursing station, frantically waving at me. I pulled up a chair, sat next to her and began trying to understand what she wanted.

It was a very interesting and challenging interaction for me. Zelda was not able to say more than one or two words at a time and the frequency and timing of her responses were quite delayed. Sometimes the words were broken or garbled, leaving me further from rather than closer to understanding what she was trying to communicate. Each time I tried to move things along by guessing what she wanted, Zelda became frantically insistent again. When I noticed myself distracted by weeding through my feelings of impatience and frustration, I realized that in order to try to meet her need I had no choice but to stay silent—inwardly and outwardly.

Zelda motioned with her crooked yet very powerful index finger for me to push her wheel chair, and off we went. She guided me to the pictures on the wall, then to various windows, then to other persons on the unit. I gave up trying to figure out what she wanted and began sharing my impressions of each thing she pointed out on our trip together. Zelda gently smiled with each comment, nodded her head and motioned us forward. We eventually returned to her position near the nursing station. I thanked Zelda for our time together. I told her that she had certainly helped me to slow down and appreciate the moment, but that I wasn't exactly sure I had really figured out what she needed. Zelda actively nodded her head "Yes" and very slowly and distinctly said:

"With...........nice...........being with."

Zelda taught me that listening in silence—*being with*—*is* an active stance. In order to be with her, it took conscious effort from me to relax my own worries, fears, thoughts and insecurities and to give full attention to whatever Zelda was presenting in the moment. I had to choose to breathe deeply and soothe my impatience with her lengthy word-finding efforts. I had to form a conscious intention to openly honor our time and take in the core of each moment she was sharing with me. Getting comfortable with the silence, allowing our relationship to unfold and joining Zelda in her world were very active processes for me.

Zelda had the present moment only. Each moment itself was full of life and was the only point where our connection could occur. By getting myself to a calm place of feeling no concern about results and of opening to being in a loving state, I could fully focus on *being with* her in her/our moment. By being willing to *be with* her, I acknowledged Zelda as a person worth my time—a person of worth. This, alone, is a powerful validating action. We were sharing the rhythm of human connection—it was a connection that was good for both of us.

Many care persons and professionals still ask, "But what can we DO?" I dare to suggest that *being with* the person who has dementia in a loving presence might be entirely what is needed in the moment. It certainly is the best way to begin. The question is a valid one, however. Frequently, something very concrete is going on for the person with dementia that distracts him or prevents him from connecting with you in that moment. Some form of intervention may be needed and it is often very difficult to understand how to enter his perception of his world in a given moment. There are four skills to be aware of in the management of silence—four tools of *being with*—that are important to discuss in detail: Touch, Observation as a Bridge, Encouraging the Person's Expressions and Listening Beyond Words.

THE FOUR TOOLS OF
"BEING WITH"

#1 - Touch

No one denies that humans need to touch and be touched. Just *Google* the topic: you will find an armload of research on adults that shows touch to have an impressive impact on one's sense of well-being and overall health. Touch relaxes, reassures, comforts, helps to decrease stress and pain, decreases anxiety, leads to positive attitude changes and is associated with happiness and vitality. I have seen persons with dementia respond to touch in all of these positive ways. More importantly, I have found that touch is a powerful and efficient way for the person to experience connection—with you, with the moment, with his past and with the expanded field of energy—that realm we call the other side, heaven or spirit.

CONNECTION WITH YOU

DOUGLAS

Douglas was a quiet man, confined to his own inner world for a number of reasons. He had been living with Alzheimer's disease for ten years when I met him at a skilled care facility. He was legally blind and "deaf as a doorknob," as he once said. Douglas spent most of each day in the resident lounge where he sat in his wheelchair, expressionless and rocking back and forth. He had no disruptive behaviors or apparent needs. Nothing seemed to interrupt his constant motion or alter his empty gaze.

One day, I brought Douglas into a discussion group I was facilitating. He was, of course, unable to actively participate in the topic of our discussion, but I figured I could at least hold his hand as a way to include him during the group. Halfway through the session, another resident called out, "Look! He's looking at you!" When I turned my head to look, Douglas was slowly reaching out to me. I helped his hand find my face and he gently traced my hair, eyes, nose and lips with his fingers. Then he firmly squeezed my hand and held it high, shaking it and smiling from ear to ear. We continued our connection through the squeezing and shaking of our hands and the joyous smile and laughter.

Human touch offers the opportunity for instant connection—the person with dementia connects with you *and* you with him. Touch is nurturing and offers safety. It is a particularly powerful way to create mutual connection with the person who has dementia and with the institutionalized elderly, since these persons tend to be particularly touch-starved individuals.

CONNECTION WITH THE MOMENT

GLADYS

Gladys was simply frantic one rainy afternoon. Her eyes were wide open, full of panic and looking at something that seemed a thousand miles off. I remember seeing that thousand-mile stare during my crisis-intervention work. She was experiencing something I could not see, that was powerfully real and traumatic for her. Gladys held onto my hand for dear life but that did not give her any discernable relief from her frightening world. I faced Gladys as she clutched my hand, trying to get eye contact to bring her back into the moment with me. She could not be diverted. Then, I tried a classic crisis-intervention technique a friend and colleague had mentioned to me just days earlier. I gently touched the outside of her knee and called her name. Gladys instantly looked right at me. I moved my hand to her upper arm/shoulder and gently said, "Hi, Gladys," to acknowledge our first connection in that moment. She began to cry, expressing the emotions that were still freshly with her. This time, however, she was not alone. I could offer her companionship, a listening ear, appropriate reassurances and human connection.

At times, the person with dementia experiences isolation, loneliness, maybe fear. Touch has the power to help that person come into a safer, more nurturing and more comforting moment—into the present moment with you.

CONNECTION WITH THE PAST

HELEN

Helen had had several transient ischemic attacks (TIAs or so-called mini-strokes) which left her totally dependent on her family and care professionals. Bless her heart though, she maintained her verbal ability. She frequently misused words and often just made up a word to rhythmically fill a space. For the most part, her sentences were incomplete bits. Yet, as long as there was a person with her who was willing and able to keep up the dialogue, Helen kept on talking.

During one of my visits with Helen, she reached out and stroked my hair with a tender and exquisitely loving expression on her face. I never saw her as beautiful as she was in that moment. I wasn't sure what she was saying as she stroked my hair. She appeared to be recapping an event from a bygone time. I responded with surprise at her more declarative statements, laughter at her humorous expressions and compassion at her more somber reflections. Her expression of love was unbelievably powerful.

At one point, I reached out to Helen and tenderly stroked her hair, reflecting the love that she had generously given me. In that moment, Helen began to talk about memories from her childhood—her words more appropriate, her sentences more complete. She told me how her mother used to stroke her hair and give her hugs and say, "You done good, little one." She shared about friendships and family and how she learned from her mother how to "give love to everyone around." She told me about the messages of kindness and generosity that she "deliberately gave to the children." At the end, Helen relaxed back in her chair and said, "I done good, didn't I?"

Touch can bring the person with dementia back to pleasant memories—a positive sensation of loving touch from a significant person in the past. This can then lead her to reminiscing and entering a life review which can then lead to her experiencing the significance of her life. Life review is an important process toward the end of life and I discuss it in more detail in Chapter 7.

CONNECTION WITH THE EXPANDED FIELD OF ENERGY

CRAIG

Craig had severe dementia. He was bed-ridden, his arms and legs were tightly contracted and he only responded to uncomfortable stimuli. His eyes had been closed for years, and according to his son, they were fully clouded over with cataracts. One afternoon, as I was gently holding his arm, Craig raised his head, opened his eyes wide and gazed at the upper right corner of his room. A look of great peace and comfort washed over his face and he lifted his head to try to see more closely what he was experiencing. He let out a series of comforting "Oh" sounds in response to the beauty that was clearly capturing his attention. Then he gently lay back on the pillow and maintained a very relaxed, gentle, loving expression. His face was thoroughly transformed from that moment forward.

NOREEN

Noreen did not want to talk with me during our visits. Instead, she motioned me to sit next to her, held both of my hands and said, "Listen to that beautiful music. You always bring such beautiful music." She said that she never heard music quite like that before—"Peaceful....calming....precious." I wasn't bringing in any music, however. The symphony of sounds was not something I was hearing or experiencing in those moments. The music was being played solely for her.

JUDY

In conjunction with Judy's mild dementia, she had other medical issues that were causing significant pain. As the nurses were trying to adjust the medication regimen to effectively meet her need, I sat with her in a calming presence and with touch. She asked me to put my hands over her abdomen where her pain was the most agonizing.

Instantly, she said she felt "God's love." Her pain left and never returned. The pain medications were discontinued, as they were no longer necessary.

Each of these persons experienced something that was beyond our usual explanations and rationalizations. Each person experienced something that was undeniably healing to them. Each showed or expressed having been blessed with a connection to something beyond the norm in their everyday, human interactions. Their experiences were transformative for them as well as for me as a witness. We all experienced entering a very sacred space that was beyond what each of us individually brought into those moments.

I encourage you to entertain the possibility that a connection through touch can be so potent that something beneficial can occur that is far greater than you can comprehend. *We all have this potential in our touch.* Of course, this thought is not anything new. Tim Harper, in *The Uncommon Touch*, discusses how the therapeutic power of touch has been used from the earliest of times. Every known world culture, from ancient times to present-day, has included individuals who used a sacred or healing touch as a medium for helping to create a more balanced state of being.

We live in an extraordinary time because such ancient knowledge is being reintroduced into modern everyday lives and interactions. Discussions and examples of consciously interacting with the healing properties of the expanded field of energy, what some call the other side or the spirit plane, are now mainstream television. Seminars and trainings in various hands-on healing modalities and disciplines are very easy to find. At minimum, to be conscious of having a loving touch and to observe whatever changes might occur with that touch will add depth and power to your connections with persons who have dementia.

CHECKING OUT RECEPTIVITY TO TOUCH

The so-called simple act of touch, therefore, helps connect the person with dementia to you, to the moment and to his past. Touch also has the potential to connect him to the expanded field of energy, which can transmit unseen healing energies. This is great! It is important, however, to keep in mind that not everyone is immediately receptive to being touched and not every moment is conducive to touching.

There are certainly cultural, familial and individual variances in receptivity to touch. Some persons have fear, repulsion, or panic-reactions to touch, because they were inappropriately touched in the past. For YOUR safety certainly, it is not wise to get close enough to touch a person who is swinging, scratching or throwing things! It is always important to check out each person's receptivity to being touched during your interactions. Here are some helpful thoughts to checking it out with a person who has dementia:

- Ask him for permission—he *always* retains the right to choose and his potential to be able to express his preferences is always present.
- If you see no signs of his permission, you can get a sense of his

openness to touch by holding your hand a few inches away from his hand or arm, for example—some place within his visual range and near a part of his body that he can move away from your hand, if he chooses—a functioning arm or hand, for example. Notice if he pulls his hand or arm away or if his eyes give a cautious look toward your hand as it approaches. This quite probably is an indication that touch is not OK for him at that time. I have known several persons with advanced dementia who were still capable of pulling away from being touched. It is important to honor each person's preference.

- Always approach the person with dementia in full view so he can see that you are about to touch him on the arm or hand. Surprise is never a good thing, in my experience. Let him know verbally that you are about to touch him and where, if he is not responsive. We always need to assume he understands and to give him permission to not accept our touch, in whatever ways he can communicate this.

- Certainly, take note of information provided by family or friends about the person's cultural history and mores or their perception of the person's unique history in relation to touch. I do suggest that you just tuck this information away as a part of the exploration, though. I have found that the family's historical perception of the person with dementia often does not match his current needs, particularly as the disease progresses. At times, our own moments with the person who has dementia are the first times in his life that he can open to the opportunity of connecting with others through a loving touch. Once again, do your own check-outs in your moments with the person and pay attention to his direct and subtle responses.

Checking out someone's receptivity to being touched means paying very close attention to his nonverbal reactions to being touched, particularly as his ability to verbalize dwindles. He might appear to just melt into your hand as you approach him with touch, or he may pull away. His rate of breathing might be interspersed with deep, comforting sighs, which could signal comfort and relaxation. On the other hand, it might become more irregular or rapid, which might indicate increased agitation or anxiety. His heart rate may shift in ways that help identify his experience and reactions to your touch. All this highlights the importance of the second tool of *being with* the person who has dementia—your observational skills.

#2 - Observation as a Bridge

Our responsibility is to somehow bridge the connection gap that widens as the person with dementia loses his ability to connect with us in familiar ways. As we are being present with him during moments of silence, we have the perfect opportunity to explore signs or clues that can tell us what he is experiencing in that moment. These clues of his emotional experience within his world are often very clear, but most of us don't know what they are and are not used to looking for them. By remaining aware of these clues of his experience and by trying to join him in his world for that moment, we actively bridge the gap between the two of us and increase the chances for a connection. These clues come from observing the person with dementia, from observing what is going on in his environment and from observing what "lights his fire," makes him happy.

CLUES ABOUT THE PERSON'S EXPERIENCE

In Chapter 2, I encouraged you to take a moment to check out how you feel in the moments just before entering an interaction with the person who has dementia and to bring particular focus to relieving any frustrations or tensions that will interfere with connecting. One reason for this is that your body has its own language and it tells everyone exactly what is going on inside you, particularly if you are distracted. This is also accurate for the person with dementia, since he forgets the social rules for hiding his inner processes and authenticity. I have found that the person with dementia very actively shows signs of his inner experience, although they are admittedly very subtle and difficult to interpret at times. I credit the extraordinary nurses at the Hospice and Palliative Care of Connecticut for helping me to pay attention and validate all of those little signs.

MR. GOLD

Mr. Gold was definitely a character. He had a very profitable business career, over 48 years of loving his wife and children and grandchildren who were committed to supporting his staying in his home for the remainder of his life. Mr. Gold loved to flirt. He enjoyed laughing at women's comments, holding their hands and flirting with his eyes long after his verbal ability faded. Eventually, he didn't speak many words at all. His eyes would just twinkle.

On one visit, however, Mr. Gold was much less active than usual. In fact, he was in bed, which was very unusual for him during the day. His privately hired aide said that he refused breakfast, which was also very unusual for him and he fought when she tried to get him up and dressed. His eyes were opened as I approached—no smiles or acknowledgments to my greeting that day. His coloring was a bit pale yet not out of the ordinary for him. His rate and pattern of breathing was normal as was his heart rate. I held his hand that was nearest to me as was our usual pattern, but Mr. Gold did not squeeze it. I said I would just sit in quiet with him, since he didn't seem to feel well that day if that was OK with him. He did not respond in any way. He just glanced at me every now and then while remaining totally expressionless.

After several minutes, I noticed that Mr. Gold was repeating a pattern with his eye movements. Each time he looked up and glanced at me, he then moved his eyes toward the opposite side of the bed and looked down. I finally told him that I was going to pull the covers back because I thought he wanted me to see something. When I did I saw that his entire right arm was swollen up to the shoulder; it was red and warm to the touch. As I reached to touch it, Mr. Gold widened his eyes which clearly let me know that he was experiencing pain and that I needed to be gentle. I called and found out that Mr. Gold was to get a visit later in the afternoon from his hospice nurse so I just left her an updating message about my observations. I also let the aide, the daughter and Mr. Gold know that the nurse would be following up later in the day.

When I followed-up later, I learned that the hospice nurse had brought the swelling down by propping a few pillows under Mr. Gold's arm. What a simple intervention and one that, if I had spoken directly with the nurse or a nursing supervisor right away, I could have easily performed myself. I could have relieved his pain and discomfort hours earlier.

I learned very clearly that it is important to notify the person's nurse of any changes I observe as soon as possible. Our observations make us an important part of the care team. In taking the time to *be with*, we may be able to observe the subtle clues more easily. The nurses are critical to the care team's brainstorming of interventions to provide the best care for the person with dementia. They will also help us understand more about the person's disease process if interventions are not effective in altering the symptom.

Some of the physical signs of a person's experience are his facial expressions, where he holds tension in his body, his breathing pattern and heart rate, his vocal quality and pattern of speech, a particular odor about him, his body movements, the temperatures and moisture of his skin, his coloring, sounds of congestion with inhaling or exhaling and body swelling. The person might be hungry or thirsty, or need a particular medication, a position change or incontinence care. Any number of things could be affecting him.

Addressing whatever physical symptom you observe will most often take priority over being in the rhythm of human connection. By helping to take care of the person's physical needs in a timely way, you will become one of the people who helped meet his very basic needs. This alone, can help begin to develop a trusting bond between you and the person with dementia, on whatever level that is possible. Your connection will be off to a very good start.

SOPHIA

The various signs you observe while being present with the person who has dementia can also clearly indicate her emotional, social or spiritual experience at the moment. Sophia had a two-year history of mini-strokes that left her with some short- and long-term memory loss. Then at age 72, after a more severe stroke which dramatically limited her ability to speak, she was admitted to our skilled care facility.

Before I greeted her at the main entrance on her first day, I observed Sophia from a distance, just to look for clues to what she might be feeling. Did she have any particular expression that indicated a mood? Was she fidgeting or otherwise in constant movement? Were any of her muscles tense? Was her respiration relaxed and deep or rapidly paced and shallow? It only takes a few seconds for this important, conscious focus each time you approach a person with dementia.

Sophia actually looked very calm as she sat in the reception area, checking out all the people coming and going. She occasionally nodded and smiled; at one point, she played with a little puppy that was being signed in as a visitor for the residents upstairs. Sophia was showing signs of contentment and happiness.

Imagine my surprise when I said, "Hi. My name is Nancy," and Sophia turned red with panic. She wailed, her chest heaving between screams as she flailed, frantically trying to hide under her coat that had been folded in her lap.

Many staff from various disciplines throughout the facility tried over the next hour-plus to help Sophia. The only thing that calmed her was leaving her alone. Only then did she return to her calm, contented state.

Our dilemma was how to help her upstairs to her unit and help her move into her room without setting her off. We tried calming words and reassurances—after all, we really weren't bad people. We tried explanations and, yes, even some bribery (that puppy she liked was upstairs where we were trying to encourage her to be). Every one of our attempts put her back into that horrible state. We pulled together a multilevel team of care professionals from the facility to problem-solve. We vented many feelings and opinions, but what were we going to do?

A maintenance worker, Trudy, had been replacing some tile in the foyer during those frightful hours and watched everything unfold. She patiently listened to all of the experiences, frustrations and theories we needed to express in our effort to help Sophia. Trudy finally said, "You know, the only time she gets upset is when you speak to her. So maybe you shouldn't say anything!" We all looked at each other and shrugged. If Trudy thought she could make it work, we said in a kind of self-humoring and challenging way, then let's watch and learn. Well, darned if Trudy didn't pantomime her way into charming Sophia into letting Trudy help her acclimate to the unit. Our avenue to connecting became clear—to explore all the nonverbal ways we can *be with* and communicate with Sophia.

As I approached my next meeting with Sophia, she clutched the arms of her chair, her respiration became more rapid, and she began to flush red. I did, after all, have this history of speaking. I established eye contact and mimed the zipping of my lips and the throwing away of that invisible key as my promise not to talk. I motioned to ask if I could sit near her and she reluctantly nodded in agreement. I sat next to her as if we were two girlfriends on the front porch in silent parallel presence. At one point I began to mirror her rapid breathing in an effort to experience more of what she might be feeling. My matching Sophia's or any other person's breathing pattern is a subtle—not obvious—technique. The other person need not be aware of what I am doing. The purpose is for me to more closely experience what the other person might be experiencing, in order to help bridge a connection. As I sat there breathing rapidly, I remembered times in my life when I felt anxious or nervous—certainly not a comfortable feeling.

Once I observed my discomfort, I took a long, deep breath to help let it go and to create a shift toward breathing at a slower, more relaxed pace. I tried to identify with what Sophia's experience must be like. She was a woman who was "Ms. Sociability, in her day," her family told me. How terrifying it must be for her—not knowing what to say or how to say it any more. I felt compassion for her struggle and with each breath I focused more intensely on taking in compassion with each inhale, letting it fill my heart, and then breathing out compassion. Within a few minutes, I noticed Sophia's breathing pattern was matching mine! We exchanged a look and a smile. A connection began.

We all learned how to use fewer and simpler words when speaking to Sophia, and how not to appeal to reason because she seemed no longer capable of being rational. We learned to focus first on fully paying attention to what was going on around her and what she was nonverbally telling us before we jumped into a moment with her. Whenever we respected Sophia's need for silence, she was open, respectful, playful and loving in connection. Her reactions helped us find a comfort zone with fewer words.

Touch also became an essential way of connecting with Sophia. Her daughter described her as a "huggie, touchie, kissie kind of mom," and we learned eventually that no truer words could describe Sophia. With the worry about verbal interaction out of the way, Sophia expressed herself freely in ways most familiar and still accessible to her—connecting to others through touch. Being with her was an experience of having your hand held and kissed, having your face lovingly caressed and getting the greatest hugs on earth! She was such a dramatically different person—more of her true self—when we were able to honor where she was at that time. She eventually was able to hear others talk to her without getting upset, but never tried to say another word. She didn't have to. We understood.

In those moments of holding our inner and outer silence, the best care for the person with dementia centers around each of us watching for the signs and clues that indicate the person's experience and sharing these observations with others on the person's care team. This is a part of actively *being with* a person who has dementia.

CLUES FROM THE ENVIRONMENT

Observing the environment offers a wealth of clues as to what the person with dementia might be experiencing in that moment. The person's ability to process outside stimuli changes as the disease progresses. He becomes less able to make sense of the world outside—discernment becomes inaccessible. All information is taken in as his senses allow, but interpretation and judgment are no longer what they once were. The impact of the environment on the person with dementia, however, remains very real and can be observed even when the dementia is profound.

LAWRENCE

Lawrence was 96 and had been nonverbal and essentially bedridden for over two years. The staff at the skilled care facility reported that he had been responsive only to uncomfortable stimuli for a year. When I entered his room one day, I noticed that his face was red, his hands were tightened into fists (not his norm) and his respiration was rapid. There was a lot of noise coming from the television. It was the Jerry Springer Show—people screaming over each other, someone sleeping with someone else's whatever and lots of bleeping. I turned it off and started playing one of Lawrence's favorites—some Benny Goodman music on a CD his daughter provided. I sat next to his bed, consciously providing a calming presence and I gently held his hands. Within two minutes, his coloring returned to normal, his hands relaxed and his breathing became calm. Was he responding to his environment? Yes, of course he was—in both cases.

MRS. TROMBLEY

At times, it takes a bit more detective work to try to unearth how the environment might be having a negative impact on the person with dementia. Mrs. Trombley had been living with her son, Edward, in his Victorian home for six years following her initial diagnosis of Alzheimer's. Her care needs had been relatively simple until recently, according to Edward. "Now she's waking up on and off through the night, screaming 'Earthquake!!!'" he said. "A few weeks ago, it was only once or twice in the middle of the night, but now it is happening from the time she goes to bed to when I get her up in the morning." Edward was exhausted, frustrated and looking for any guidance we could provide.

Before resorting to sleeping medication, Edward wanted to explore alternatives to helping his mother sleep through the night. We talked about the progression of his mother's disease and how it was affecting her perception of her environment. We brainstormed about what could be different in or outside her room at this point in time, as opposed to a few weeks ago.

Edward decided he was going to sit up all night, if he had to, to pay very close attention to every detail around the situation. We constructed a log for him to record his observations—space to write the time of night that she screamed, space to record observations about his mother, space for observations about the environment and space for notes about what helped her get back to sleep. As I was leaving, he was in search of a hat and pipe to "complete the Sherlock experience." I am still not really sure if he was serious about that, however, the thought tickled me.

Two days later, an elated Edward called. On that first night, he sat in his mother's room as she slept. It took three or four times until he discovered that his mother was awakening with the sound of the old furnace going on in the basement directly beneath her bedroom! The nights were getting much colder with winter rapidly approaching, so the furnace had been firing up more frequently. "Whenever the old dinosaur fires up, the whole room shakes and rumbles—Mother thinks it's an earthquake!" Edward moved his mother's bedroom furniture into a different room on the first floor, farther away from the furnace. She slept through the night. Edward said, "The Case of the Irksome Earthquake" was closed.

To the person with dementia, the world outside does not make the same sense it did in the past. Shadows against the curtain may be seen as a person trying to break into the home, rather than a result of the street light shining through the trees at night. The people on the television or radio are actually in the room and the person with dementia often feels responsible for holding up her end of the conversation or for "offering them a proper cup of tea." Lines on the floor can be perceived as steps, spots as pieces of garbage that need to be picked up. The person with dementia lives in that moment she perceives and progressively loses the ability of discernment she once possessed.

Because of this change, we need to observe the environment with different eyes. It is important to try to really see what is going on around the person with dementia as if we were looking at the environment for the first time, without any past associations or assumptions. Watch and pay attention in silence during those moments of *being with* the person who has dementia. You'll discover amazing ways to simplify things to make the environment more nurturing and supportive. *The Complete Guide to Alzheimer's-Proofing Your Home* by M. L. Warner is a useful resource full of ideas for creating a safe and workable home environment. There are also several other resources listed in the back of this book that include many suggestions on changing the environment as the disease progresses.

CLUES FROM 'WHAT LIGHTS HER FIRE'

While we are being present with both inner and outer silence, we have an opportunity to expand our observations beyond the difficulties or the things that are apparently going "wrong" with the person who has dementia. We also have great opportunity to closely watch for clues as to what sparks her—what helps light up her enthusiasm and joy in connection. At times, it appears that not the slightest ember could possibly be left after the disease has run its course. Still, I am constantly surprised at how the flames can be rekindled when we pay close attention.

ADELE

I visited Adele every week. At 93, she was living in a skilled care facility under hospice care for her advanced dementia. Each week I sat next to her bed, where she always lay very peacefully with eyes closed and hands gently interlaced on top of her abdomen. I always introduced myself and asked permission to spend time with her—no response ever returned. Occasionally, I asked permission to hold Adele's hand (no response), but she most definitely pushed my hand away as I reached out each time! OK, touch wasn't her thing. Her respiration did become deeper as I sat with her and her heart shifted to a slower rate than when I first entered the room each time. At least this was some indication that I was having a positive impact as I sat in calm and loving silence. I kept visiting.

On the 7th-week visit, Adele was in the same position as always. I had long since stopped asking her if I could hold her hand and had explored many other ways to connect—all to no avail. On this visit, for some unexplainable reason, I began to hum a tune that popped into my head. I looked over at Adele. Not a muscle in her body moved except in her face, which shifted into a full scowl! "Oh, fine!" I said, "a critic!" With that, one side of Adele's mouth turned up into a little smile and she began to hum in a very soft, high, frail voice.

From that time on, Adele and I had a humming relationship that pleased us both immensely. I would start the humming, she responded with her humming, and we went back and forth for our entire time together. Humming was the path for Adele, to reentering the joys of human connection.

ROZ

Roz was in deep grief during her first weeks in the skilled-care facility. She was still able to put thoughts and words together—certainly in a different pattern and with unique wording, but she was actively communicating some basic ideas. The losses of her home and self-sufficiency had unearthed all the powerful losses she had endured through-out her life—her parents' and husband's deaths, her "stupid decision not to have children" and unfulfilled dreams. As I lis-tened to her tell her life story over many visits, I looked for clues as to what were her strengths and joys in life. One day, I entered her room for our regular visit and Roz was watch-ing a baseball game on the television. I encouraged her to keep the game on so we could share it together—after all, this was the first interest in anything she had shown since her admis-sion. At one point, she very sadly said, "Man…a beer. That's all I really need—baseball and a beer, you know?" I casually said that I could see if the doctor would prescribe a beer for her. Suddenly, Roz looked at me with the wide eyes and gap-ing grin of a kid in a chocolate factory. "You COULD!?" That suggestion certainly hit the spot! I explained that I knew she didn't have a history of alcohol abuse, but I wasn't sure about mixing alcohol with her medication. I told her that was why I had to consult the doctor.

Well, the doctor wrote a prescription for one beer a day and that one beer totally transformed Roz's way of being in her new world. She was right—a beer with her base-ball game was all she really needed. It empowered her to regain a sense of control over her life and her ability to enjoy and participate in life. In a period of two years at the facility, Roz emerged from a state of total isolation into being president of the resident's counsel.

LINDA

At times we have to ask family and friends for clues about what might spark joy for the person with dementia. One of the most surprising leads I received was from Linda's granddaughter. Linda had moderate dementia when she fell and broke her hip. It appeared that the surgery "tipped her scales," as the doctor phrased it—she never talked or opened her eyes after that. There seemed to be a lot going on inside Linda's head, however, because throughout the year following her surgery, she had facial expressions that convinced us that she was having active encounters in her inner world. Yet none of us could figure out how to access that place with her.

I asked her granddaughter about her memories and knowledge of Linda's past; what she most enjoyed in life, what were her strengths. Instantly, her granddaughter said, "Hands down—Hawaiian music!" Linda's access to her best coping and to her playful and joyful side had always been Hawaiian music. I must say I would never have guessed that one. Well, lo and behold, when we played a tape of Hawaiian music in her room, she opened her eyes, looked at us all smiling at her and said in a rather surprised way, "Well, Hello!" Linda was back—still very confused of course, but now open to reconnecting with others around her.

While *being with* a person who has dementia during moments of silence, we have an opportunity to look closely for various clues that will help the two of us connect. Persons with dementia have taught me that it requires a stretching outside our traditional boxes. The person's "spark" might be her love of music or dance. She might connect powerfully with others or with her Higher Power in the form of religious rituals. (It always stunned me how Roma could perfectly recite the prayers over the candles at Oneg Shabbat yet could not put any other coherent thoughts together the rest of the week.) She might most powerfully connect through the use of humor or with puppets. The list of possible pathways into connection is open-ended.

#3 - Encouraging the Person's Expressions

It is the verbal and nonverbal expressions of her experience that help our ability to *be with* the person who has dementia in her world, from her perspective. Listening in a way that encourages her to express what she is experiencing in the moment is an active stance. Here are a few ways we can actively encourage her expressions with our calm presence, body posture and words.

OUR CALMING PRESENCE

The more calm, open and relaxed I am during an interaction with a person who has dementia, the more she is able to express herself. All of us have more difficulty pulling our thoughts together and expressing ourselves when we are experiencing tense or difficult feelings as opposed to when we are in a calm place. The same is true for the person with dementia—even more so!

ROSIE

Rosie had been a grade-school science teacher for 40 years, and she had recently been diagnosed with Alzheimer's disease when I met her. She said that whenever she got upset, her thoughts and feelings "get thrown into a large pot, all scattered about and it's impossible to do anything with them, like those tiny little metal filings."When someone gets upset with her she said,"Their filings go into the pot, too—what a mess!" She loved talking with me, she said "because your quiet calm is like a magnet; it pulls everything into alignment and lets me speak clearly."

Rosie's experience underscores the importance of relaxing your opinions and judgments, opening your heart and keeping an inner silence. As the person's ability to relate her experiences decreases, we all too rapidly become hyper-dependent on our brain power as we try hard to understand the mismatched or nonsensical details. We spend too much time sifting through the scattered metal filings trying to mold them into forms that make sense to us. We spend so much effort translating, interpreting and puzzle-solving, that we exhaust ourselves and get frustrated if our efforts don't apparently help. Our frustration and fatigue then add to everyone's confusion and interfere with the person's full potential for expression.

A very critical practice therefore, is listening with a quiet mind and a feeling heart. Remember to breathe. Center and calm yourself before entering each new moment with the person who has dementia. Breathe into and through the heart; feel its rhythm, and bring your attention on keeping it open with love. This will help pull you away from your analytical thoughts and settle you into stillness or inner silence. It will help do the same for the person with dementia, if only on that powerful level of energetic communication between the hearts.

Consider this possibility as well: as you focus on your own open and feeling heart, you might be able to connect directly with the nonverbal emotional experience of the person with dementia. This kind of focus encourages or exercises your inner knowing—your intuitive sense—which often leads to the successful intervention that your logical mind has been unable to bring about. I will spend some more time exploring intuition in Chapter 7.

OUR OPEN BODY STANCE

When my body language says, "I am interested in what you have to say," then my mere physical presence is powerfully effective in *being with* persons who have dementia. There are several ways my body communicates interest: I show it when I make eye contact with the person who has dementia, to the extent that he is comfortable with eye contact. I face him directly and lean forward slightly so that we are at eye level; if I haven't checked my tense and closed body positions at the door, I relax and release them before I go any further. I nod my head in response to his verbalizations and because I am interested, my facial expressions show my interest in what he is saying and communicate to him that I am paying full attention. I sit calmly and allow him enough time to express himself.

Our bodies can also mirror the physical rhythms of the person with dementia in such a way that we communicate that we are actively there *being with* him. You might have an opportunity as I did with Sophia (page 123) to get in sync with the rhythm and pattern of his breathing to try to get a better sense of his experience. You can also walk with him while matching his stride, steps and sway. You might gently rock with him as he rocks in place or move in whatever way mirrors his body language. Your face, too, can reflect his. This allows him to possibly see and better identify the feelings you see in his facial expressions. All of this mirroring, of course, is not done in an obvious or dramatic way, which he could perceive as mocking. These body reflections are to help you better experience the other person's world while communicating that you are *being with* him.

Touch is another physical action that can bring us together on levels probably more numerous than we can ever know. As stated before, the person with dementia certainly has greater potential for knowing I am with him if I am holding his hand or touching his shoulder. I can also use touch to let him know that I am really listening to what he is trying to say or express. As he is talking, I might reach out compassionately to support or reassure him. A gentle squeezing of his hand or arm indicates I will continue to listen, that I understand what he is saying, that he is not alone... any number of things. Touch can also open my heart so that I am able to listen in a different way.

OUR ENCOURAGING WORDS

We certainly have no problem listening to the person with dementia when his words and expressions make sense to us. However, for those times when words skip or dance unpredictably and the communication seems foggy, here are some concrete ways you can verbally encourage the person with dementia to continue sharing his world from his perspective:

- You might occasionally ask a question that will clarify something the person is saying. Getting *his* facts by asking the basic *who, what, where, when, why* can facilitate him telling his story; it can help clarify and give you a better understanding of his truth. Since his ability to verbalize is often quite limited, you can ask simple questions that require only a simple yes or no—or just a few words—to answer. Here's the caveat: too many questions can come across like an interrogation. To avoid putting him on the defensive, observe his verbal and nonverbal clues. Stop your questions if he is irritated by them or continue if it appears that he feels supported by them. Let him be the guide.

- Use the same words or phrases that she is using to tell her story; a calm and gentle loving tone is usually best. At other times, using her words while reflecting her tone of voice can be encouraging. This says to her that you are listening to her words and that you are paying good attention. It also honors her way of saying whatever she needs to say and encourages her to continue.

- Repeat his expressions or thoughts to help him stay on track with the thoughts he is trying to communicate. The person with dementia usually greatly appreciates this, since keeping a train of thought is a significant challenge as the disease progresses and particularly when he is upset about something. It also, once again, shows you are listening and you want him to continue.

- Giving some positive feedback along the way is also powerful encouragement. The person who has dementia is all too familiar with feeling put-down and ignored. You can, for example, let her know when she is effectively telling her story or communicating a point. You can thank her for being patient with your difficulty in understanding at times; this takes the blame off of her. You can help her understand that her gift to you is allowing you to share this time with her (more about this in the next chapter).

There are many ways and opportunities to encourage the person with dementia to be more expressive. As you try these and discover others, remind yourself often to take it easy and resist judging yourself harshly. In the beginning, the goal is to pay a bit more attention to the verbal and nonverbal ways that you present yourself to the person with dementia. As you do this, as you notice what you bring into the room, you will also take in the variety of responses the person with dementia will have to you. Remember, to listen effectively, try to keep an inner silence and consciously stay in your heart. With this as your home base, the rest will just flow.

#4 - Listening Beyond the Words

As a social rule, we listen with a focus on the words in order to understand what others are saying. During interactions with the person who has dementia, listening in that way is a challenge, at best. This fourth tool for *being with* suggests that our concept of listening needs to expand, that to be with the person who has dementia requires a different way of listening.

For one thing, active listening to the person with dementia will take more time than casual or ordinary listening. He needs time to sort through the jumbled bits of his thoughts to express what he is trying to share. We need to give ourselves time to try to understand his communications and his experience.

The number one interference in allowing more time is our fix-it mentality—the tendency to jump into problem-solving mode. This cuts off the person's expressions prematurely and denies his right to have a voice. As we bounce through our guesses about interventions, he can often feel invalidated or even more isolated. Sometimes he blossoms into full-blown frustration or rage or simply recoils into himself. Putting the fix-it impulse on hold creates more time for us to understand and validate his experience.

Our new way of listening is not about grasping content but about allowing the unfolding of and our identifying with the experience of the person with dementia. It is about you understanding his reality and truth without judgment. At times you might feel as if you are in a foreign country. This is actually not a bad correlation. The person with dementia often speaks in what sounds like a foreign tongue; he is frequently in a different time zone and dimension, operating from points of reference which are unfamiliar to you. As is true when you travel, when you take time to acclimate to the environment and negotiate the new territory, you begin to understand how to communicate with others. You need to give yourself permission to allow the slow revelation of the other person's experience and to honor it with patience.

THE LISTENING STRETCH

As access to words and concepts becomes less available to the person with dementia, our listening to her messages has to stretch proportionately. Her ability to find words and pull together thoughts becomes less straightforward as the disease progresses. What we hear is often unclear, emotionally charged and takes us further from understanding her world than when we first approached her. But how does this marry with the concept I mentioned earlier—that the person with dementia is always authentic, that how she presents is exactly who she is? Although her words and thoughts are not straightforward to us, she continues to express her emotional experience. Her ability to cover up her emotions diminishes.

In listening to her perceptions therefore, you must relax your habit of listening for linear word-by-word declarations. Her ability to put thoughts and words together becomes increasingly inadequate, rendering her verbal messages only clues to her actual experience. Your way into understanding her experience is to broaden your listening into hearing themes, concepts and significant words that stand out in her expressions. These will help you navigate the sea of confusion so that you can hear and respond to her underlying emotional experience.

As you begin to hear themes and significant words in the verbal expressions of the person with dementia, you simultaneously open to listening to yourself. It's almost automatic. As you remain open to that personal experience, you gain opportunity to fully enter the moment with the person who has dementia. As you begin to hear certain themes and to identify her emotions, as she expresses them both verbally and nonverbally, you can direct your attention inside yourself to see if you can empathize. Were there times in your life when you experienced similar feelings? When we can truly see and accept the person's feelings as real and human, and reflect that to her, she will feel cared about and "seen." We will be validating her as a person of worth. Transformation becomes possible. Perhaps it is easier at this point to give examples of persons who have entered my life and helped me learn how to accomplish what I've just described. I have chosen five persons who represent different emotional states. I will share each story up to the point of our connection and the shift to a balanced or calming interaction. Later in this chapter, I will continue each story and show how each person and I, in this more balanced and connected state, were able to move forward to more effectively problem-solve and create some surprisingly long-term transformations.

Note that with each person, I began by consciously breathing to release any of my own tensions and emotional baggage, so that I could open my heart to entering the present moment with loving consciousness. If I became tense, frustrated or distracted, I practiced deep breathing to bring myself back to the moment and to the reminder to breathe loving into my heart.

Expressions of Sadness, Emptiness, Loss

JULIA

Julia's words made incrementally less sense as each year passed, but she always maintained a sense of playfulness and joy. She was an absolute favorite on the unit where she had lived for four years. She loved to sit "out and about all the action," as she used to say. However, on one particular day she showed all the signs of a sadness—a down-turned mouth and eyes, slow and soft vocal qualities, watery eyes, a more flattened affect and her hand over her heart. I was called to the unit to see if I could find out what was wrong.

I sat down facing her at eye level, reached over with a gentle touch on her hand and said, "Julia. You look so very sad. What's going on?"

Her eyes stayed focused on the floor as she said, "I miss my tezerish."

"You miss it?" I used the word that I understood, that communicated the most to me about her experience. The "missing" was the point. I chose the ambiguous "it" to refer to the word that didn't make sense to me. It really wasn't about what specifically she was missing at this point—it was that she was having an experience of missing, of loss and sadness. To dwell on "tezerish" would have been to skip over her emotion, which was being clearly communicated in nonverbal ways.

"Yes," Julia said. There was a long pause as her tears streamed down her cheeks. I continued to hold the silence to give her more time to respond, all the while giving compassionate hums and squeezing her hand at times to support and to encourage. "Why do daskob treap off?" she said after a while. The theme of loss—of having been left—seemed to stand out, once again.

"I'm not sure why." This was an authentic answer, which I followed with a silent pause. "Can you tell me more about what went off?" I gave her the time to express what appeared to be some of her memories of "daskob," encouraging her with all the listening skills. She frequently used key words like "love," "beautiful," and "important" interspersed among her jumbled words and sentences. Successive statements didn't really clarify the words I didn't understand; however, the themes of missing or of questioning would continue to surface. Her eyes never left their focus on the floor in front of her.

As she talked, I heard these key words and themes and let them help me listen to her story from her perspective. Her key words or themes showed that she so dearly loved someone or something that she was missing. I could certainly identify with the experience of dearly missing someone with whom I was strongly connected. On that emotional level, Julia and I had a bond. I leaned closer to her and said, "Julia, I don't know exactly what you are missing, but I do know what it is like to miss something that I love. I'm so sorry you have to feel such sadness."

With that, Julia instantly looked up and established very long and connected eye contact with me. It was clear to me that she felt totally heard—no longer alone in her sadness. We were walking together in that moment. We exchanged compassionate, loving smiles with each other—a very powerful moment for both of us.

Expressions of Confusion, Searching, Feeling Lost

MR. DONOVAN

"Where did the goshing doodle fig? Where? Doodle fig, doodle fig!" Mr. Donovan reemphasized, as if that would help me understand what he was talking about. "Fast!…fast!" His eyes were darting down the hallways, his arms waving for dramatically descriptive clarity. He showed all the nonverbal signs of someone on an urgent quest—the questioning eye brows, eyes trying to find the target, walking about in an increasingly frantic search. As he hunted, his words became more confused and louder. Perhaps he hoped such emphasis would add to the clarity. It didn't. He became more frustrated.

Sitting and talking was not what this interaction was going to be about. It was clear that to *be with* Mr. Donovan I had to go with him on the hunt. I said that I did not know where "it" was, but that I would help him look for it, if that was OK with him. He reluctantly nodded in agreement, giving me a doubting look, possibly questioning my motives. We set off on our quest, looking into every room, every corner, on every unit in the building.

As we were walking and searching, I could identify with his frustration. I was a bit frustrated with being unable to help solve his problem—to find whatever he was seeking. I also thought of the crazed frustration I felt earlier in the week when I was searching for my house keys and the overwhelming concern that I must be going insane when I finally found them in the freezer! Those were not happy moments! My compassion for this man grew as we continued our search.

When Mr. Donovan exhausted himself and all the avenues of searching, we went back to his unit where he sat down in a chair. His expression turned to one of confusion, his eyes more questioningly moving about as if he was trying to sort out mismatched pieces of information. I sat down in front of him, put my hand on his arm and sincerely apologized for not being able to find what he was looking for. I added, "It is so confusing and frustrating for me when I can't find something...makes me feel like I'm going crazy!" With that, Mr. Donovan raised his head, looked straight into my eyes, and said with a unique clarity, "Yeah...but I'm so glad you tried."

It was clear to me in that moment, that he felt his feelings were validated—by my words at the end of our journey as well as with my action of staying with him throughout the process. His response was astonishingly clear, articulate and stated with a loving smile. I was deeply moved by the sincerity expressed in his words and eyes. Until that moment, I was not even certain that he was aware of my accompanying him on this journey. I no longer had any doubt.

Expressions of Fear, Vulnerability

LENORA

On my first morning back from a vacation, I was called to an emergency team meeting. The discussion regarded changes in Lenora, whose daughter described as "always having been a very calm, even-keeled woman with 102 years of amazing history." Throughout her life she had shown "only loving, never difficult emotions"—she was her family's "tower of strength," even as her dementia progressed. Unfortunately, Lenora had a very difficult week. The team felt that she was living a different nightmare every afternoon and they were frantically searching for something that would help her.

The team informed me that one afternoon in the area near the nursing station, Lenora began rapidly shaking her head, and calling out, "No.....sign, sign, sign.....not,

not....no!" Another day she was rocking back and forth, arms crossed over her chest tightly, saying, "Don't... kitaliff...stop; stop...kitaliff!" Each day, she spoke different words, but her body language, the panicked expression on her face and the urgency in her voice all clearly communicated fear and a sense of vulnerability. They said that the only thing that helped was taking her to her room and spending time with her alone.

We still couldn't figure out what was causing her to panic each day.

The only similarity in the episodes of emotional upsets that the team could see was time of day: they always occurred in the early afternoon.

That afternoon, the team paged me. Lenora had been taken to her room, but this time remained in a panicked state, saying, "I didn't, I didn't......no, no....can't go, can't go.....stop!" As I entered the room, her widened eyes darted toward me, she recoiled in a defensive posture and her hands were shaking dramatically. "No.....NO!....can't go!" I immediately said— very calmly, softly, yet in a firm, reassuring voice— "Lenora. It's me. Nancy. I'm here to stay with you and we'll figure out what's going on. I'll make sure nothing happens to you, OK?" With that she reached out for my hand and clung onto it, rapidly kissing it and holding it to her cheek. This approach clearly let her know that she was not alone and that I was there to help her. It was essential to try to immediately address her fear with a calming voice and with reassurance.

It is never appropriate to try to convince a person with dementia that her experience is not real. Of course it is real. This is *her* world and *her* reality! We are explorers! To debate as to whose reality is correct would be to lock each of us into our separate worlds. Lenora had reasons for feeling the way she did—how outrageous it would have been for me to try to tell her how she should feel! My position was not to deny her reality, but to try to help her express her perceptions and her feelings about her experiences in that moment. Perhaps I could also get some clues for future problem-solving, and minimize her fear episodes each afternoon.

While still holding her hand (she was never going to release that grip!), I continued to use her words saying, "Lenora, you can't go where?" She talked and talked, much of it not understandable and in partial statements. The words that were repeatedly stated were "jail" and "cave," her body gestures mimed being scrunched into a very small space. The theme was always in the words "can't go" or saying she "didn't." I eventually asked her if she was afraid someone was going to lock her up in jail, to which she said, "YES!" She began to breathe more rapidly and shake again. I asked her to look at me, which she did. I said very sincerely, "Lenora, if someone was going to lock *me* away, I'd be pretty scared myself! And if someone is going to try to lock *you* away, you better believe they will have to go through me first!!! I can get pretty scrappy, you know!"

At my telling her I identified with her feelings, and my reassuring her with strength and a touch of humor that I would protect her, Lenora wrapped her arms around my neck and hugged me, repeatedly saying, "Love, love, love, love…" She totally transformed from the previous moment and remained calm and loving the rest of the day. Later in this chapter, I will return to Lenora's story to show how future episodes were averted.

Expressions of Anxiety, Worry

MRS. GARNER

"Someone…help me!" were the words that echoed down the hall as I first walked onto the unit one afternoon. "Help me, PLEASE!" It was Mrs. Garner, working very hard at pushing the wheels on her chair forward, her eyes desperately searching for a care professional. When I reached her, I squatted down to talk with her at eye level and asked what she needed. "I have to go pick up my children! Please…can you help me? They're at school and it's time to pick them up. I have to get there right away. Please help me!"

By asking some very basic questions, I understood that she was definitely talking about her children who were, in her perception of that moment, ages six, seven and nine— "Way too young to be left alone in the school yard! I need to pick them up! Please help me get there!" She was right about it being 3 PM and school letting out. I asked the names of her children and what they were like. I asked some questions about parenting three children so close in age, seeing if I could try to shift her attention very gradually away from her determined focus. She had no time to humor me and said with some irritation, "What does that have to do with anything, anyway? I'm worried about my children!"

OK. Distraction wasn't going to work! That was clear.

In the previous examples, the stretch for me was to relax the way I listened to the words that were being expressed. With Mrs. Garner, the stretch in listening for me was to relax my need to talk with her in *my* time frame and to be willing to enter *her* time frame in order to understand her experience. This was a woman who was worried about her responsibility for her children—not a light concern. Trying to convince her that they were the grown up adults in *my* time frame would be both inappropriate and ineffective. She knew what she knew. I thought about the times I was worried about my children and their safety. It is a horrible, helpless feeling to not be able to get to them, when you believe they need help.

Plan B: I told Mrs. Garner that I have two children and I certainly know what it is like to worry about them. She was instantly relieved and grabbed my hand and said, "Then, will you help me? Please tell me what to do." I told her that I would ask around to see if anyone left a message about the children—"Maybe someone else is picking them up today or they're playing over at a friend's house?" She paused for a moment and thought.

"If Girtie picked them up she would have certainly told me!" I told her I would ask around and let her know as soon as possible. Mrs. Garner was comforted for the moment and stopped calling out, feeling reassured that I was researching the issue.

I went to the nursing station and talked with the staff. They had already tried everything they could think of to help calm Mrs. Garner. They even got her daughter on the phone to have her tell her mother that she was fine. Mrs. Garner just said, "Who was that old lady. I'm not stupid, you know!" My hope was that enough time would go by while I was talking with staff that Mrs. Garner would forget her focus. After all, she was much calmer now that she knew I was taking her concern more seriously. Unfortunately, each time I looked up and toward Mrs. Garner, her eyes were glued at me. She was clearly anticipating my return and the resolve to my search. OK. Forgetting her focus wasn't going to happen on that day!

Plan C: I returned to Mrs. Garner and she immediately said, "So, what did you find out?" I decided that this was one of those moments that called for some truth-stretching: "I just picked up my messages and there was one from Girtie. She picked up your children today. They are fine. I'm so sorry I didn't find out sooner and that you had to suffer all of this time, Mrs. Garner." The part about my being sorry that she had to suffer was, of course, very heartfelt and sincere. I communicated the message with very direct eye contact and with the reinforcement of a compassionate, hugging touch on her arm.

Mrs. Garner remained a bit irritated for a while, but as we sat together in silence, her shoulders relaxed to their normal position, her hands gently folded into themselves, and her breathing turned into deep sighs of relief. Very gradually, we shifted toward a lengthy conversation, beginning with the worries of motherhood and ending with more joyful memories and with her children's accomplishments. I reflected to her that I was sure her children were wonderful people because she was such a concerned, loving mother to them (all quite sincere and truthful—from conversations and interactions with her adult children over time, I knew them to be wonderful people!). She glowed and returned such a loving look at me, saying: "Come on, honey…time for a big hug!"

Expressions of Anger, Blame, Accusation

GARY

Let's go back to Gary (Chapter 4, page 98), the 78-year-old man whose dementia had progressed to the extent that he was endangered in the community. A judge had appointed Gary's son to be his conservator. By the time he first entered the extended care facility, Gary's rage was elevated to an art form. His anger and blame brought everyone's blood to a boil, as he spit out obscenities and accusations at us for our ignorance, stupidity and collusion in conspiracy against him. He lashed out with arms swinging and throwing anything he could find at any one of us who said something he didn't want to hear. If that didn't get to us, he would go for the more personal touches and degrade some body part or mannerism that was most often each person's deepest insecurity.

Our very human reactions were to become angry in return, either inwardly or outwardly. We became angry and frustrated that Gary wasn't hearing *our* perspective. From our perspective, he was acting crazy and irrational. The irony is that he was feeling the same about us. We weren't listening to *his* perspective either, and we clearly must be "the crazy ones" if we didn't believe what he was telling us. From his perspective, he was "the only sane one in the bunch!" We were locked into our separate worlds. So how could we bridge this huge gap?

I was clear that a warm, fuzzy smile at this time would, at best, certainly not have reflected where he was in that moment, would not have been authentic of me and probably would have fueled his flames. Before entering the room, I was aware that a part of my 'stretching' was to take time to prepare myself for the anger that Gary would express toward me and the feelings this might generate in me. I had to remind myself to try to let go of such emotions as hurt or anger because this is Gary's *disease*— not Gary. I needed to enter that interaction with openness to hearing Gary's perspective in that moment, without prejudgments or expectations. I needed to breathe into and through my heart.

As I knocked on the door and began to enter the room, a chair flew across the floor. Clearly getting close enough to provide calming, reassuring touch wasn't the choice in this moment! I said to him in a firm voice, "OK. I got the message. You're angry!"

"NO S__T, YOU BRAINLESS B____H!" GET THE F___K OUTA HERE!"

Well, the good news is that I had spent several years living in a girl's dormitory. That form of expressing oneself wasn't really foreign to me, or threatening, if you know what I mean. Still, it didn't feel good. I took a deep breath to let my reactions go. Gary was right about one thing; his anger would have been obvious even to the numbest species. So, I agreed with Gary that it didn't take a rocket scientist to figure out that he was angry, but that I seriously wasn't clear as to what his anger was about. "I want to understand YOUR thoughts, YOUR take on this." I matched his passion while emphasizing the specific words.

The most important step was to spend time listening to Gary's perspective on what was happening. To do this, my active focus needed to be on my inner silence, since he was particularly adept at finding people's buttons. I also took the stance of an investigative reporter, asking *who, what, where, when, why*, while using as much of his own wording as possible. I watched for signs of irritation, which could indicate that my questioning was too much. I provided a lot of 'air time' to allow him to talk and to vent. I listened, paying full attention to his perspective and leaving my opinions and judgments about his behavior and his dementia outside the door. It was important, in that moment, to try to fully enter his world with open and genuine respectfulness.

"You think you want my story? I'll tell you my story!!!" he screamed, as he continued to yell it for the next 45 minutes. During that time, I learned that I had to stretch beyond my need to hear logical conclusions and facts. To really look at the situation from Gary's perspective meant, of course, that he *was* the only sane one. He was "still young" (only 32 years old in that moment) and was quite an accomplished artist. His home was also his studio, where he had, for over 40 years, built up quite a following in the art community. His sculptures were displayed in cities around the nation, he told me. "How can they rip me from my work?"

Gary had no memory of any problems: his walking out into the streets in sub-zero temperatures without a coat or shoes, his getting lost trying to find his way home from the grocery store down the street, his forgetting to eat and take his medication. His son's and the care professional's attempts to convince him that these problems existed had seriously failed. To Gary, there was "no reason for being in this place."

As I listened, focusing on putting myself into Gary's position, I wondered how I would feel if my only reality was what he presented. I very honestly, genuinely and in his same passionate tone of voice said, "Gary, I've gotta tell you. If people in my life were trying to rip me from my work, I'd be furious, too. I really would." Gary stopped and held a long silence while he searched my eyes for sincerity. He knew in those few moments, that he had been heard. His demeanor completely changed and he eventually said in a softened tone, "What the hell is your name?"

"Nancy."

"Nancy, what the hell am I supposed to do about it?" He was beginning to trust me *and* elicit my help in solving his dilemma.

"We'll have to figure out what to do about it together, Gary...if you'll let me help, that is."

With that, he nodded and said, "Well, let's hurry it up!" The story of our evolving connection continues in the next section of this chapter.

MOVING BEYOND

As we enter each moment with the person who has dementia, we can adopt a new receptivity and go beyond our own boundaries of memories of the past and anticipations of the future. The person is your best guide to her experience in any given moment and you can encourage her to lead you if you have an open heart and use inviting gestures, both verbal and non-verbal. The intention is to find the essential emotion within her story, and respond in relation to her truth about her world, in that moment, on that day.

Once you identify her emotion, find ways to empathize with that feeling. To empathize successfully, focus on her emotion and not merely on the facts as she presents them. Minimize your tendency to analyze and interpret the details; it is simply inappropriate to do so, as is debate or disagreement with her truth. To dig too deeply into or to challenge the facts or details of what she is saying, keeps both of you in separate versions of reality and locks out any hope of a connection. The person with dementia believes the reasons for her feelings and her need for self-expression is valid. That's enough.

Allowing yourself to temporarily identify with the experience of the person with dementia, and see it from her perspective is an essential way into a connection. Can you be with *her* truth and take it in, even for a moment, as if it were your own? In her article entitled "Valuing Vulnerability," Judith Jordan says there is an "as if" quality to empathy, a *trying-on* willingness, in which we place ourselves in the other's shoes. Can you recognize parts of yourself and how you approach the world in what the other person is expressing? Would you feel even a little of what she is feeling, in the same situation? Have you ever experienced similar feelings? These places are where your worlds overlap, and where you can find a connection.

Identifying with some aspect of the emotional experience of the person with dementia, even in a small way, gets us across that gap that separates us. To be authentic, as Jordan points out, we do not have to totally disclose our life story, or all the specific details about our identification with the other person's experience. Nor does it mean that we dwell in it, so that we are bonding in our common miseries. Our authenticity lies in our ability to be fully present with the person who has dementia in a real, responsive way, and to let her see her real impact on us.

Reflecting our identification with her lets her know that she was heard and that she is not alone. By "reflecting," I mean telling the person some aspect of what we related to in her expressions. Our emotions may overlap in this instance. While it is never accurate to say "I know how you feel,"—in my opinion, because we could not possibly know all the aspects of how a person with dementia feels in all the ways the disease plays out for her— we can authentically relate and respond to some aspect of her experience. We then find ourselves standing on the same turf, on the same side of the connection gap, where we have greater opportunities to enter the rhythm of human connection.

There is a mutual quality to *being with*, as J. Surrey points out in her article entitled "Self in Relation." One side of *being with* means that the other person is *being seen* by me and that she *feels seen*. As the above examples show, however, there comes a turning point during the interaction, when the person with dementia clearly sees me too, and I feel seen by her. We both feel the power of those connecting moments and this mutual connection moves us forward. As J.B. Miller identifies in her article, "What Do We Mean by Relationships?," each of us feels a greater sense of worth and increased vitality and energy. Each of us gains a more accurate picture of her/himself and of the other person. Each of us feels a powerful connection with each other as well as a greater motivation for creating connections with other people. We both are more able to act, without getting stuck in a communication gap.

Let's go back to continue each person's story and see how they moved beyond their stuck place with the power of meaningful connectedness.

Julia's Sadness Transformed

Julia and I took our time enjoying our very long and connected eye contact, our exchange of smiles and handholding. I eventually said that I wasn't totally sure what she was missing, but that "sometimes it just plain makes us feel better to be with someone else when we are feeling sad." I asked Julia if she would like me to stay with her for a while and she rapidly and with a lot of animation said, "Oh, yes!"

My being with Julia helped bring back her sense of playfulness and joy. She began to notice the action going on around her, nodding and greeting staff and residents passing by. We walked around the unit and shared comments about the art on the walls, laughing at those which may have required, shall I say, a more sophisticated level of art appreciation than we held. Along the way, we involved other residents in three-way conversations and shared the joy in those moments. We eventually stopped by the recreation center and talked with the recreational therapist about activities that might interest Julia.

In an attempt to try to shake up some widely accepted misconceptions, I need to underscore the fact that recreational activities have the potential of going far beyond the entertainment value or a *just-keep-them-busy* mentality. A well-designed recreation program offers a profoundly therapeutic component for the person with dementia. A major part of the emotional difficulty that comes with the disease stems from the person having nothing to do.

During her entire life, she has been an involved, productive, useful, contributing human being but with the onset of dementia, she is often suddenly treated as though her usefulness to the world around her no longer exists. There is nothing farther from the truth! Good therapeutic recreational programming meets each individual's very human need to remain involved, useful and productive. In group settings, this supports the person's need for connection in community. She feels valuable and valued.

Giving Julia something to do and the opportunity to be part of a group helped support the shift she had begun by connecting with me. The recreation therapist knew that Julia had a history of loving colors and crafts projects. Fall was rapidly approaching and the therapist was thinking of ways to encourage residents to participate in decorating Julia's unit with visual representations of the new season. At this, Julia's eyes lit up and she eagerly began to work on the project. She took the next step in her shift toward becoming reinvolved with the world around her.

Mr. Donovan's Confusion Transformed

It amazed me to see how clear Mr. Donovan became after we established that initial, strong connection. My helping him search the facility for something dear that was lost to him, even though it was unidentified to me, created trust between us and the opportunity for a connection. After a long pause of being with each other nonverbally, he stood, reached for my hand, and we were off to his room. He went to the dresser, picked up a picture of his daughter, pointed to it and said, "Where?" That was certainly very clear! I asked if he was wondering where his daughter was. He said, "Yes!"

I went to the nursing station and called his daughter to find out. She said that she had just popped in briefly to "say hi" to her father, but had left without saying good-bye. Unfortunately, many family members make a practice of not letting their loved one know they are going—*Please Don't!* The rationale is usually one of two unpleasant beliefs: (1) "Dad always forgets when I come to see him, anyway," and (2) "It is always so hard to leave him…I feel so guilty." In reference to the first point, I have found that the person with dementia, as was true with Mr. Donovan, most often does remember when someone he loves has visited, at least in the immediate time frame. When he is left without being told, he often feels a sense of loss. Not remembering why he feels sad or empty, he may not be able to effectively communicate his feelings. Families can help by always communicating with care providers when they were visiting and when they are leaving, to help take the guesswork out of moods that later surface in the person with dementia.

In reference to the second point, it *is* often difficult to leave the person with dementia, particularly if he pleads with us to stay and keep him company. I have found a few things to be helpful. I asked Mr. Donovan's daughter to seek my assistance (or that of other care providers) to help with leaving. Care providers can catch him up and stay with him to help offset the separation. A great help for Mr. Donovan was that his daughter put up a calendar on which she logged when she visited and when she would be returning. When she would be away for longer than a few days, she left cards in his room or mailed them. This kept open the lines of connection between the two of them. The staff read the cards and reinforced the information on the calendar to Mr. Donovan each day. This helped him feel secure in his daughter's ongoing involvement in his life.

As each intervention was created and reinforced, Mr. Donovan no longer entered those highly confusing, searching places. He became more interactive with other residents and found a wonderful role as the "soother" of his unit. Whenever anyone was particularly upset, Mr. Donovan pulled up a chair next to her and gently patted her hand to show his support. He was very effective in helping to calm the difficult feelings of five specific residents. Few words were ever spoken—it was his purity in *being with* each one.

Lenora's Fears Transformed

Lenora was calmed by my immediate, calming, reassuring voice letting her know that I took her feelings seriously, heard her messages and would protect her from what she feared in that moment—being taken to jail. She easily shifted toward interacting with me. Lenora began to introduce me to her family via pictures that I had seen so many times in the past years. She reclaimed her gracious hostess skills and offered me some chocolate from a delicate, lidded china bowl, saying with pride, "It's been in the family for years, you know." "The chocolate?" I asked with a teasing smile. "Oh, no. This little dish. Now take a piece of chocolate, dear." Of course, I wouldn't think of disappointing her! Lenora and I were back into a connected rhythm, once again. The fearful episode was no longer a part of her reality. What a joy to see.

The dilemma still remained as to what was causing her to have these experiences each day. It was important to see if there was some way to avoid these very upsetting episodes for Lenora in the future. Our team reconvened and we, once again, went over everything that occurred on the unit before the episodes occurred. The nursing staff strongly felt that a consultation with the facility's psychiatrist would help. They believed that Lenora might be having hallucinations of some form that could be eased with medication.

Since the psychiatrist was not due in for a few more days, I decided that the next day I would go up on her unit early in the afternoon and commit my main focus on observing how the afternoon ensued for and around Lenora—perhaps there would be some other clues that the team couldn't notice while performing their heavily paced tasks. I sat behind the nursing station, fielding some phone calls and doing some paperwork as I focused most of my observations on the unit and Lenora's reactions. The team also became hyper-vigilant—all of us invested in trying to solve this mystery.

All of a sudden, it happened. Lenora screamed out, "THE LIONS......DON'T EAT, DON'T EAT!!!" At the same moment, the entire team that was present turned and noticed that the afternoon oldies movie playing on the television was a circus movie. The lion tamer was inside the cage working with three, very hungry lions. Even though Lenora was not looking at the movie, she was paying active attention to the plot as it was unfolding to her ears. Lenora could no longer differentiate between her own reality and what was playing out on the television set. She became a part of the action and her life was being threatened just as much as the lion tamer's.

That was the glorious afternoon that the team finally agreed that the television at the nursing station was, indeed, not a good thing. It was removed immediately. Lenora's pattern of fear in the afternoon was interrupted—without the use of medication. She lived out the rest of her years without ever again returning to that fearful place and staying in loving connection with all who entered her life.

Mrs. Garner's Anxiety Transformed

Certainly a part of Mrs. Garner's shift away from her distress about her children getting picked up from school came from feeling that her concern was taken seriously. She was simply relieved that I was going to help solve her dilemma and reassured that her children were safe. While this did help resolve the crisis of the moment, however, it was not enough to completely open her to enter into a connection with me (or anyone else). It was the conversation that followed that helped her continue to relax and fully shift toward the potential for connection.

A part of the effectiveness of my conversation with Mrs. Garner was my awareness of the importance of reminiscing. By asking questions and entering a dialogue with Mrs. Garner about those early memories, I could help her verbalize all of her worries and feelings of being overwhelmed with the responsibilities and burdens of motherhood that she was clearly working through. I could also gradually shift the conversation toward a more positive focus by asking questions that explored the other side of the equation, such as asking her if it was *always* hard for her as a mother. Mrs. Garner shifted into the fond, loving memories of the truly remarkable children she raised. When I reflected this back to her, she fully acknowledged the connection we made in those moments.

With the crisis ended, once again, problem-solving with the team needed to try to shift this three p.m. turmoil that Mrs. Garner felt almost every day. We figured two factors were at work: it was both the time her children had historically been let out of school and it was shift-change time for facility staff, dependably chaotic every day. We decided that an essential part of helping Mrs. Garner to decrease her anxiety level each day would be to give her something to do. We heard that she was feeling as though she had responsibilities she was not able to perform, so we decided that perhaps giving her a responsibility that she could perform each afternoon might help in some way.

During part of our conversation, I asked Mrs. Garner if there was anything she used to do that helped calm her whenever she became worried about something. She said, "Solitaire...helps me sort it all out." Mrs. Garner's daughter also told us that she was a lifetime card player—you name it: Canasta, Bridge, Poker and Gin Rummy. It really didn't matter. Mrs. Garner loved all card games. She no longer remembered how to play them, but we found that she loved to move cards around and to sort them. So, at 2:30 every afternoon, the team set her up at a table in the lounge area and gave her five jumbled up decks of cards to sort out and to put in order. She loved it. She was helping the recreational therapist keep her cards in order each day and was performing a task that she both excelled in and thoroughly enjoyed.

Mrs. Garner returned to feeling like a responsible adult and to feeling good about herself, even as her dementia continued to progress. Giving the person with dementia something to do that includes a consideration of her lifelong interests or best coping skills, often diverts difficult times and helps her feel more like a person still capable of participating in life. The 'doing' may be a concrete task, as was true for Mrs. Garner, or it may be an enjoyable activity. Sometimes, a part of 'the doing' is in simply being with other persons and connecting in the ways she can. The key is to explore how she has coped with difficult times throughout life and to support connections with those coping skills that will help her as she is trying to adapt to her ever-changing world.

Gary's Anger Transformed

I first got Gary's attention when I authentically acknowledged that I would have strong feelings "…if people in my life were trying to rip me from my work." He not only knew I heard what he was upset about, but he also heard my validation of his feelings. This diffused a major piece of his anger. A connection with Gary began in that moment.

Moving forward with Gary required more of his story. I asked him to tell me more about his son, who he had labeled the "enemy," the "Gestapo," the "warden." He vented about how controlling and pushy his son was—"He has no respect any more." "Any more?," I asked, leading him to reminisce about what their relationship used to be like. Gary leaned back into his chair and talked at length about how his son used to have great respect for him. He talked about the days of teaching his son how to fly fish and how to build his own labyrinth behind his home. Gary's son used to go to him for guidance and advice on practically everything. He had no idea "what happened to those times…it wasn't like it was all that long ago, either."

I said that it just didn't make sense that his son would change into such a totally different person so suddenly and asked him if it would be alright with him if I did some more research about it, to get a fuller picture. Gary tensed up and shouted, "They're going to tell you I'm CRAZY!" I calmly yet passionately said, "I already KNOW you're NOT crazy, Gary. You do need to know, though, that right now you don't have any rights. The only way out of here and to live as independently as possible is to go back through the system that put you here."

I went on to say that I have to find out all the reasons why he was brought to the facility and why his rights were taken away by the judge and given to his son. I explained all the steps necessary to get a doctor's evaluation and to successfully overturn any decision in the courts. I also talked about other living environments that might be suitable for him, and that choosing any such alternatives would require a doctor's evaluation. "It's a pretty big labyrinth, Gary," I said. "Since I've been through it before, I am just asking if you would like me to walk through it with you." I deliberately used "labyrinth," of course, because this was a word he used in connection with his son—I knew he would identify with it.

Gary agreed. I needed to make a deal first, however. I said that I would commit to taking the time to research all the information, brainstorm with him about what options to explore, and advocate for him wherever possible. I also said that I, as well as the other care providers, would promise to treat him with the respect that he deserves. In return, I wanted his promise that he would treat me and the other care providers in a respectful way. This was defined as no name calling and no throwing objects of any kind.

"I don't know if I want to do that," he said, thinking out loud.

I just kept looking at him and held the silence. He needed to come to it in his own time. Finally he stood. "You drive a hard bargain."

We shook hands on the deal. I wrote it up in contract form, signed by us all. It was a great memory tool for him and we could all refer to it when needed.

Gary remained grumpy, stubborn and demanding—this, his son told us, had always been his M.O. He did go through the process with me, though. A part of my focus was to check out whether this really was the best placement for him and to present to him the variety of considerations for his review. Each day, I gave him an update of my progress—which person I was waiting to hear from or which meeting or evaluation was being scheduled.

Another part of my immediate focus was working on setting up his environment to better suit his needs for whatever time he was to remain at the facility. There needed to be some constructive outlet for his creative energy, which had been his most functional coping skill throughout life. We recreated his room and another space in the facility to support his work. Changing his environment to support his artistic interests was a relatively immediate shift that both supported his best lifelong coping mechanisms and helped support trust-building. Movement was occurring for him—things were getting better in bits and pieces.

In the five months that followed, a lot did happen. With the supervision of medication and the provision of regular nutrition, Gary's condition improved to the point where the doctor stated that he qualified to move to more of an assisted living environment. I worked with Gary and his son on the healing of their relationship and they toured various facilities that would allow Gary more freedom yet provide him with enough supervision for his safety. The doctor did not feel Gary had the judgment to be able to live on his own at this point in his disease process. Gary never accepted this analysis, of course, but on some level he knew it was accurate. He eventually made the decision to stay at our facility, rather than "up-heaving everything and moving to some other dump." As he put it, "You never know what will happen in the future. Besides, I like being the sharpest tack in the box."

That was the day Gary gave me the sponge chair he made for me to throw back at him (Chapter 4, page 98). That was the first day that we saw him smile. Gary was able to move beyond his stuck place when we dared to cross over that bridge into his world and to try to see it from his perspective. By the way, this shift was another example of progress achieved without the use of additional medication.

SUMMARY

Marge Schneider, a good friend of mine and author of *A Hand in Healing: The Power of Expressive Puppetry,* told me that I certainly have a lot to say about not saying so much! A great many people do not yet understand or trust that there is rich experience and potential inherent in silence and in the art of *being with* a person who has dementia. Our distancing reactions, confusion, defensive challenging and judgments have a direct impact on persons with dementia. One person might withdraw so deeply that it becomes very difficult for us to break through the isolation. Another might become powerfully locked into his emotional state and hold desperately to his reality in order to keep a sane self-image. So much of this disconnection can be bridged by our openly exploring the potential of silence.

Being with the person who has dementia is not about merely staying in the person's presence, being nice and giving him a forum for talking or just hanging out (not that there's anything wrong with that, you understand!). *Being with* the person with dementia is your opportunity to remain outwardly and inwardly silent, so that you can hear and enter the truth of his experience, however it plays out. In open silence, you can identify and listen to the emotional truth that the person with dementia needs to express. By being available you get the extraordinary chance to really see, accept and empathize without judgment, and to validate the emotions and the person. Regardless of how isolated or distanced he seems, when you explore by accepting the guidance of the person with dementia, your mutual abilities to enter the rhythm of human connection has more of a chance to ignite.

The examples in this chapter highlight the multidimensional and, at times, very challenging nature of this level of *being with*. I want to also emphasize that the opposite is simultaneously true—that connecting with a person who has dementia can be very easy. With the slightest shift in your approach, you will see how easily your interactions with most persons who have dementia will transform. Your smallest gestures can shine amazingly and like a bright light, draw the person into connection.

I saw a great deal of evidence of this during my years as a social worker in extended-care facilities.

My position as a social worker was often defined by the team as "doing everything that no one else wants to do." I rather preferred to say that we social workers provided the grease to help all the gears in the facility operate smoothly. Whatever the framework, my daily reality was most often running from Crisis A to Crisis B, passing by (give or take) 15 residents sitting out by one of the nursing stations. I learned to wear clothing that flowed, creating the visual of grace and beauty as I moved by them. I waved at individuals, gave a huge smile, laughed at my crazy day, complimented a hairdo or a piece of clothing, blew kisses and at times did a little "Shuffle Off to Buffalo" on the way through their unit.

To you and me, I did an endless list of little silly things. To these persons, I made little connections that left smiles on faces, created laughter and brought bits of joy and connection in those moments. It is extraordinary, the power of the simple gesture!

With even the smallest of connections, I tried to pay attention to how each person responded and to what was and was not effective, allowing myself to make adjustments to better meet the person where he was in each moment. By letting him guide me into his world, I stretched beyond my own limitations into more freely expressing my playfulness and joy. I became more willing and able to be fully present and to honor each exploration toward connection. I developed a profound thankfulness for how each person helped shape me as a person in this world. I found opportunities for letting each know how he has affected my life. Initially, I had no idea that these expressions, to some, would have a dramatic impact and help to create even more unexpected shifts.

WORKING IT OUT

Expand the ability to be with others in silence.

Experience Hands-On Treatment

Schedule a hands-on treatment with a Reiki, Shiatsu or Reflexology practitioner to experience the benefits of healing touch. Try a massage or acupressure treatment. There is an entire array of hands-on healing modalities available. Only you can decide which modality and which practitioner is the best for you. In the search, begin by getting a recommendation from a person you know and respect. Perhaps check with local licensing or certification agencies or with Associated Bodywork and Massage Professionals (*www.abmp.com*). Spend some time asking about qualifications and experience. Get to know their approach to their practice. Spending time to interview the practitioner will help you see if they are in alignment with your needs and preferences.

This experience will not only help validate for you the beneficial effects of touch, it will also encourage your openness toward receiving it.

Watch a Foreign Language Channel

Judith Blahnik, my dear friend, suggests watching the Korean channel (or some channel broadcasting in a language that is foreign to you) on TV. This can be quite fun. After an overly analytical, high-intensity day at work, you may get to the place of settling into *being with* the program and feel soothed in this unknowing state. Sometimes it is very relaxing and comforting *NOT* to have to figure what's going on or get wrapped up in the details of the moment.

You also may find yourself entering the world you are observing and sense exactly what is going on with amazing clarity. You may actually become irritated. Making a mental note of possible causes of the irritation can increase your self-awareness. Perhaps it is an old, familiar gremlin...e.g., getting locked into the need to know or judgment about the program's content or about yourself. That's OK—you have the power to turn off the TV if you are not having fun. That's the best part!

Expand Your Awareness

SCHEDULE TIME FOR SILENT, MINDFUL ATTENTION

One of the best practices for me is to schedule some protected time just for me—a date with myself. I suggest the same for you. Schedule a block of time to do something by yourself that nurtures and sustains you—a block of time when you can reacquaint yourself with your true nature, when you can simply *be with* yourself. For this date, make a plan to give all your attention to something that you will thoroughly and effortlessly enjoy while being as silent as possible.

There are no rules as far as how much time to set aside for your date. Many people feel their pace is so wild that they can't even think of claiming a full day, an evening or a morning each week for themselves (although, wouldn't that be wonderful?). Perhaps only an hour a week or an evening each month is all you can cut out for yourself. Whatever you decide on, mark your calendar as you would for any other serious commitment and hold yourself to it. When you honor it in this way, I promise you that you will not be disappointed. You will also probably find it easier to plan future dates.

During your personal time, pay attention to what most opens your heart and gives you joy. Whenever your mind floats away toward the "real world" and all the waiting frenzy, gently bring your attention back to whatever you decided to focus on during your private moments. If you decide to listen to music, take it in fully and let it fill your heart. Dance, if you choose—no one is around to judge your form. If you enjoy walking, take in the beauty and magnificence that surrounds you. Notice the colors and textures, the graceful movements of the trees, creatures, smells and sounds. With each breath, take in the beauty and the blessings the awareness provides and let them fill your heart. Whatever most nurtures your body, mind and spirit is what is important to do during your date with yourself. Fully absorb the support and acknowledge how wonderful it feels.

KEEP TRACK OF THE "LITTLE HITS"

During the late 1980's, I asked Linda Keiser Mardis, my teaching Reiki Master, what I could do to expand my awareness of my more intuitive side. She suggested this:

> Get a little notepad—something very easy to carry around with you throughout the day. Every time you have a feeling or a *hit* that something is going to happen or each time you notice one of those tiny "coincidences" that occur all the time, make a note of it on your notepad. For example, you may be just thinking of a person with whom you haven't spoken in a while and he or she just happens to call on the telephone. Write it down. Or, you are standing in front of a bay of elevators and have a *hit* that the one in the middle will open first—and it does. Write it down. Or, you are thinking of something out of the blue and the person you are with brings up the same topic. Write it down. You get the idea.

This practice will do, at minimum, two things. First, it will validate for you that you really do have intuitions that are often simply explained away as coincidences. When you cluster them together and see how often this occurs, you will begin to acknowledge that you do, indeed, have an intuitive side. Secondly, paying attention to your more intuitive nature will help reinforce and strengthen it.

JOURNAL

Keeping a daily journal is one of the most effective ways to communicate with your own inner wisdom and with the wisdom of the expanded field of energy. Commit to getting up a little earlier each morning to write at least three pages. Some wisdom teachers suggest writing on focused topics, such as reflections on or insights from dreams, meditations, biblical passages or poetry. Julia Cameron, in her book *The Artist's Way*, recommends writing "morning pages," which amounts to free-form, stream of consciousness journaling designed to clear out your thoughts and emotions. Your writing may sound whiny, grumpy or petty at first, but it is a great way to give voice to those gremlins and then physically put them away. Allow the ideas and thoughts to flow without judgment— they are meant only for you, never to be revealed to others. This practice will allow you to face the day more clearly and to be more present in your life. At times, a brilliant idea or thought will float to the surface, deepening your sense of inner wisdom and the wisdom in the expanded field of energy.

6 – Thankfulness

SARA

Sara's life was a weave of tragedy, hardship and grief. Her entire family—parents, aunts, uncles, cousins, husband and children—were wiped out by the Holocaust. We learned from a close friend of hers and from a previous social worker, that she came to this country with two dresses to her name. She worked hard throughout her life, scrubbing floors to make a subsistence-level income. Sara would not remarry—she knew she could "no longer bless a marriage with children," as she had said, so she had closed herself off from relationships with men. By the time she arrived at my facility, the obvious signs of a traditional beauty had long since faded, and Sara's dementia had progressed to the point where she was totally dependent on care professionals for everything. At best, she was able to have one- or two-word interactions with others. All day long, she quietly sat in her wheelchair with hands gently folded on her lap.

We never could have predicted how being with Sara and watching her interact with her world would be an extraordinary gift. The simplest things filled her with joy. One day, a tiny spider found its way to Sara's arm and caught her attention. She gazed at that spider with childlike wonder and concentration, widening her eyes with delight each time it shifted direction. Other days, she immersed herself in the flower-pattern of her dress and traced each flower with her fingers, delicately admiring their beauty. She responded to each spoonful of the pureed food we gave her to eat with an "Mmmm" and a gentle, savoring smile. And even during very brief contact, Sara still looked deeply into the eyes of her care professional, smiled and said, "Thank you."

Sara was my guru; she taught me to open to the beauty of slowing down, and actively appreciating the world around me. I had *read* about people living a life of gratitude in works by numerous psychologists, philosophers and modern theologians; but before Sara, I had never actually *seen* it in action! None of my early role models ever slowed down because to slow down would bring on self-absorption and misery; to fully take in and appreciate my surroundings would compromise my protective barriers and the likelihood of survival. I learned, as too many of us do, to keep very busy, to be driven and to strive for perfection (whatever that is!)—certainly not to take time for reflection. The deep inner peace and attitude of gratefulness which Sara embodied and the sages discussed were so compelling to me—I wanted some of that!

My occupation, which allows me to fully participate in the life experience of persons with dementia, is an enormous blessing. The work gives me innumerable gifts. In order to connect with each person, I have to relax and be present—with my mind and my heart—in each moment. Interactions require me to be more receptive to hearing, feeling and understanding different perspectives. Each day I am taught again to stretch beyond my ordinary abilities and to watch and listen for clues to the real experience of the person with dementia. She guides me with reactions and, at times, blunt feedback to push beyond my narrow, singular perspective. As a result, I am more self-aware, more humble and much more respectful of the person with dementia and her tutelage.

As I hope the stories in this book reveal, it is the person with dementia who strengthens my ability to honor her past and appreciate her current strengths. She passes on to me some of the wisdom of her lifetime. She reveals the purity and authenticity of her emotions. When we meet on this common emotional level, I realize we both have come out of isolation.

The impact of persons with dementia on me has been at least as great as my effect on them. I have experienced two disparate realities energetically co-existing and interconnecting in relationship. Challenges become possibilities; problems give way to solutions; isolation dissolves into connection. We shift to the same rhythm—unconcerned about what the next step is. We simply allow our interactions to unfold. Details about what each of us is 'giving' or 'getting' matter less than experiencing the vibrancy in our relationship.

Each of us grows a little and feels better for having connected with the other. With each such experience with a person who has dementia, I became thankful more readily and easily. When I did, it seemed to throw a toggle switch that kept me from giving rise to anger, worry and unhappiness. The negative circuitry just could not get through. I felt filled and complete. This was a wonderful thing! It became very natural and important for me to express my appreciation to persons with dementia and the only way I knew how was to sincerely say, "Thank you." As did so many things about this work, discovering how dramatically persons with dementia absorbed my expressions of thankfulness surprised me.

THE IMPACT OF EXPRESSING THANKFULNESS

He Helped Someone Feel Good

MR. PHILLIPS

Mr. Phillips had lived at home for five years after his diagnosis of Alzheimer's disease. His wife was devoted to him and deeply committed to meeting all of his needs in their home of 52 years. She kept up with all of his incontinence care and provided constant companionship, answering the same questions a million times over. She supervised him day and night, as she feared he might walk out of the house at night as he had done once before. Of course, everything else involved in running a home still had to be done. She balanced household chores with handling finances and doing yard work for the first time in her life.

Unfortunately for her, Mrs. Phillips turned down the many offers of help that poured in from her sisters, cousins and friends. They were worried at the darkening circles under her eyes and her dizzy spells that had started happening. They tried to talk with her about their concerns, both individually and as a group, thinking "maybe one of us would get through to her." Instead of giving in, however, Mrs. Phillips refused to let them visit anymore. She didn't like them noticing those little things and challenging her ability to do it all. So, Mrs. Phillips dropped dead in the middle of one night—of a heart attack. Mr. Phillips had to be moved immediately into the skilled care facility—exactly the fate his wife was trying to prevent all those years.

To put it bluntly, Mr. Phillips did not thrive during his first three months at the facility, before our first meeting. No one was quite sure of his baseline abilities. He sat in his room all day, just staring at the wall. The psychiatrist tried to prescribe antidepressants—it was very logical that he could be in a state of depression following so many traumatic changes—but Mr. Phillips always pushed away any pills brought to him. He clenched his jaw when food was offered and survived only on nutritional supplements he accepted every day or two. He had lost 45 pounds by the time I first met him, and at 5' 10", he weighed in at 121 pounds, a number that was decreasing daily.

When I introduced myself and told him that I was there to keep him company, to spend some time with him, Mr. Phillips made no sign of having heard anything. I pulled up a chair and sat next to him for quite a while, as a calming presence. I became aware of the long spaces between his breaths. I could also see how infrequently his heart was beating, by watching a vein in his hand. I slowed down my breathing to match his, finding that I could not keep up this slower pace very long. I could only imagine where his thoughts were, yet certainly felt compassion for this man who had been through so much. So I "just" sat with him in that state of loving compassion.

I eventually asked if I could hold his hand while sitting with him. To my surprise, he opened his palm. I held his hand for about another 15 minutes in a state of calming presence. I noticed that his breathing began to pick up and his heart rate increased, both coming to match my own. His cheeks became pink and his eyes softened and began to focus on pictures displayed on the wall. I felt his hand gently squeezing mine. We had a connection! I was "with" him and he knew it; he was "with" me and I knew it. I was so genuinely touched by that moment. This dear man was able and willing to reach beyond his depression and his confusion and take the risk of connecting with me. (I say risk because opening up to connection is not always the path of least resistance.) I was so touched by our connection that I simply and sincerely said, "Thank you, Mr. Phillips."

He looked up at me with total surprise, established direct eye contact, and said "Whatever for?" I was equally surprised

both by his verbalizing any words at all and by my own immediate response of, "The gift of sharing yourself with me." Mr.
Phillips instantly broke into tears. I remained silent, allowing
space for his tears to flow while holding his hand and squeezing it occasionally for support and reassurance that I was
still with him. He turned to me, grabbed both of my hands,
and said "I didn't think I could." After a long pause he said,
"You feel good? You feel good?" I nodded and said "Yes!" He
leaned back and, with tears of joy and grief, he said, "I didn't
think I could, I didn't think I could."

The thank-you I expressed communicated to Mr. Phillips
that he was still able to have a positive impact on someone—me. Mr. Phillips clearly felt a connection *to* me when
he squeezed my hand, but he didn't have a clue that he had
such a positive effect on me until I thanked him. My artic-
ulation of thankfulness was evidence to him that he was
now in connection *with* me—it was not a one-sided relationship. As I felt good that my presence was helping him
to feel good, he felt good that he helped me to feel good.
Mr. Phillips realized that he was still capable of being in the
rhythm of connection—no longer "garbage" (as he named
it later on), no longer merely a passive receiver of another
person's kindness. He began to experience himself as a person of value. He was appreciated, wanted and useful.

From that moment on, Mr. Phillips started participating
in life again. He ate all his meals and gained weight; he
joined in recreational activities; he developed a significant
role for himself—his unit's friendly greeter. He always
wore a suit and a tie and was quite the dapper gentleman—

the ladies of the facility simply loved seeing him each day. They looked past his repetitive greetings and his continual pacing. Having someone walk by and gently wish them a pleasant day or stopping to just be with them for a while made everyone feel good.

She Engaged an Important Person

LOLLIE

"Lollie was quite the lady," her loving nephew told us. It wasn't her choice to walk the more traditional path for women in her time—to take any one of many offers of marriage and to have children. She spent her years fighting for women's rights, working as a machinist in a shipyard during the war, founding and running a downtown soup kitchen and being hostess to countless immigrants and refugees over her 94 years of life. As her nephew put it, "Lollie was a gentle, loving woman who always had a cause." With the progression of her disease, however, Lollie's cause became *Me against the world.*

Over years of living with dementia, Lollie increasingly pulled away from people. During the six weeks before our hospice team was called in to help, she became very paranoid and felt that everyone was trying to poison her or get rid of her. The only nutrients she occasionally took were milk or juice from unopened containers that she carefully inspected for needle marks with her magnifying glass. Lollie would say that she "wouldn't put it past those sneaky nurses in this place to put something in these little boxes—they're very clever, you know!" She lost 17% of her body weight in six weeks—a frighteningly rapid weight loss which, if allowed to continue, would have certainly resulted in death within a few months.

When I first walked into her room, she gave me *that look.* You know the one—the look that would have totally obliterated me in a nanosecond, if only she had perfected that laser-beam-from-the-eyes technology. She was quite animated and screamed out, "Oh, great! Another one! When are you stupid nurses going to get it that I'm not taking any of your stupid medicine! Get out of here!" I responded equally dramatically, "BELIEVE ME. YOU DON'T WANT *ME* AS A NURSE! I don't do that medicine-needle-blood thing, OK? That's why I'm just a social-worker-type-person." Luckily, she didn't hate social workers...yet. She *very* reluctantly allowed me to stay, making it clear that I was not to interrupt her program.

As I sat next to her, I noticed in my peripheral vision that Lollie was breathing very rapidly, her face was red, her heart rate elevated, her body in continually fidgeting movement. The unit nurse had told me earlier, "She's wound up and spinning like a top these last few weeks—all the time. And she won't take anything that will help her." The staff was very concerned for her. This was totally the opposite of how Lollie behaved in her former life. I was brought in to see if she could trust someone who was not employed by the facility, and to see if being with her as a calming presence would have a relaxing effect on her. Unfortunately, I could find no signs of my having any calming effect at all. Her breathing, heart rate, coloring and fidgeting remained consistent.

I looked around her room. To start at square one, for me it felt just plain good to be sitting down—it had been such a hectic day. I began to notice all the volunteer awards with her name and a picture of her standing with Eleanor Roosevelt. There was a picture of Lollie as a younger woman, playing on a beach somewhere with her three sisters, each one of them had beautiful, joyous smiles. There were many pictures of people she had obviously connected with and, no doubt, significantly helped throughout her long life of deep commitment to various missions. I welled up with a profound sense of gratitude that this woman honored the world with her work and consciousness. During a commercial break in the program, I gently leaned over and said, "Thank you, Lollie."

"ME!" she said, and she searched my eyes for the reason why she was being thanked. I told her, "It feels so good to be sitting with you right now. Thank you." "I don't understand," she said. "*You're* the hot shot! I'm nothing anymore, just ask them. I'm a confused, stupid, meaningless nothing." I asked her to hold my hand and look into my eyes, which she willingly did. I spoke in a matter of fact tone, reflecting her words back to her, "Lollie, 'hot shots' don't talk with 'nothings,' you know what I'm saying?" I have no idea why, but that made a lot of sense to her— our connection was born and a new pathway opened.

Lollie began to share with me her perceptions of her world, during which time none of the signs of her agitation went away. Actually, she appeared to become more agitated as she recapped all her evidence that she was the target of the nurses—"They're trying to kill me, you know." She wished she could trust them to give her a medication that would help—"I want to just jump out of my skin," she said. At one point, however, she stopped long enough to tell me that it felt "so good to hold someone's hand." She briefly reminisced how she used to love to be touched and to touch others. "But," she said, "I won't let these nurses touch me anymore."

I asked, "ALL of the nurses are horrible here?" "Yes," she said emphatically..."Well...all except Peggy. She's the only good one."

I spent a long time, gingerly talking with her about something that could help her feel better. I told her about how our hospice nurse told me that morning about a particular cream we could try to order for her, if she was willing to try it. This cream could help her relax more and could be massaged into her by the nurse she trusted. Lollie was very reluctant yet drawn to the idea of getting a cream massaged in—"But only by nurse Peggy, you understand...only Peggy!"

I do not usually advocate the use of medications as a first intervention. For the vast majority of persons with dementia, positive changes in difficult behaviors can be made either by shifting our approach or by making creative changes to the environment. It is important, however, to recognize that medications are not inherently evil. With the progression of dementia, the person undergoes a variety of physiological changes in the brain that affect her perception and ability to function as she once could. There are times when the person may be experiencing a chemical imbalance that is leading them to think that bugs are crawling under their skin, or that little people are telling them not to trust anyone. Sometimes they're like Lollie and want to jump out of their skin because the agitation is too intense. We can only imagine how uncomfortable and frightening such states would be. To leave them in those states when there are options that could help would be cruel.

Certain medications, used under the watchful eye of caring medical staff, are at times an excellent intervention to help rebalance or to create a positive shift for the person with dementia. Their use is not for our care professional's or care person's convenience, but for the benefit and comfort of the person with dementia. While loss of affect, animation and other responses can be side affects of medications, we cannot assume that all medications will automatically *snow* the person, as most people fear. Other risks include increased likelihood of falls, drowsiness, confusion and changes in temperament. The important focus is for the person, his care-persons and professionals and medical professionals to work together in order to observe and to make decisions as to the best course of treatment, one that will create a better overall balance for that individual.

In Lollie's situation, all alternatives failed to create for her a feeling of safety and comfort. The hospice nurses, upon physician approval, have access to some amazing compound medications that have been highly effective for persons like Lollie. The relaxing medication is added to a cream that makes possible the absorption of that medication through the skin. The massage also feels good! The sole purpose of the prescription for Lollie was to take the proverbial *edge off* the anxiety or paranoia, and to allow her to be maximally functional, once again.

It worked! Within a few days, Lollie was eating normally and regularly throwing only two specific people out of her room—"I never liked them, anyway!," she said. After a few weeks, she was participating in recreational activities again, returning to her normal weight and "back to her more sparkly self," according to her nephew. Lollie was discharged from hospice-level care. Simple words of thanks from someone whom she felt was important had been the catalyst for her open problem-solving and change.

She Effectively Communicated Her Experience

KATHYRN

I was in one of my 'flitting zones,' as I call it. I loved going through the unit where most of the moderate and severely demented persons lived, greeting and briefly making connections with 15 or so residents who were often sitting near the nurse's station. It certainly let me be highly functional, since I could do a quick check in and make corrections on all the so-called 'little things' that may have gone awry: Larry's hearing aide was missing; Freda's lap tray was slipping off; and *where* are Julie's darn glasses!? Again? As I complimented Alice's dress, I could discretely pull the hem down below her knees—my goodness, we could see all the way to France! Then I could make a call to her daughter to discuss the apparent need for Alice to switch to wearing slacks. I could give Mrs. Garner her deck of cards or Mr. Lathrop something to fold. As I said, it was a very productive time.

What I loved the most about flitting were the little connections during the briefest moments. What a thrill to see someone's eyes light up as I complimented her hair, makeup or dress. It was such a joy to share a good laugh, a smile, perhaps dance a little and be so openly playful—kind of like a pollination thing. It became quite the focused art form. With even the smallest of connections, as I mentioned at the end of the last chapter, I tried to pay attention to where each person *was* during the interactions. But, I must admit, on one particular day the art form and the fun took over my fully paying attention. Not to worry. Kathryn was there to bring me back to earth!

I was flitting around the unit in a particularly cheerful mood that day. Several of the residents were quite alert and playful. I was having more and more fun, seemingly gaining momentum as I went. Eventually I made my way to Kathryn, who was sitting in her wheel chair and who apparently had

been watching me much of the time. I gave a very enthusiastic "Hi, Kathryn! Good to see you this afternoon!" She
looked straight at me with an angry face and said, "WHAT
THE HELL ARE YOU SO PERKY FOR?" She brought me right
to the point. I realized that I was so involved in spreading good
cheer that I was not at all paying attention to the fact that
Kathryn was not in the same place that afternoon. She did-
n't want to be in that place. My agenda, if you will, was taking over. I was not being sensitive to first observing where
she was in that moment. What an extraordinary awareness
for her to bring to my attention!

In our split second greeting, I felt thankful to her for
clearly calling my attention to my insensitivity. I apologized and said, "Thank you, Kathryn. I got it…perky is not
where you are, today." "*No it's not!*" she said, still with her
anger. I reached over, pulled up a chair and sat quietly
next to her for a moment. I then, very softly said, "Thank
you so much Kathryn, for telling me so clearly." At that
moment, Kathryn's shoulders relaxed and her scowling
face turned to sadness.

My thanking her let her know she had clearly communicated her need. Now she could trust that I would be available—interested and able—to listen to her. She began to
speak about an event in the past that was upsetting to
her—a fight between her and her sister that has caused
years of distancing. With partial sentences and mismatched
words, she communicated her emotions clearly and knew
I was fully present with her. At the end, we thanked each
other for the beauty of having shared the connection from

which we both gained a lot. Ever since that day, Kathryn's face pops into my mind as a reminder to keep some consciousness about where each person is when I am in the *flitting zone*.

They Were Helpful and Useful

ALL 60 RESIDENTS

The staff of the skilled care facility went into a state of confusion and panic when we heard one Monday that on Thursday we would have to evacuate 60 residents to another part of the facility so that repairs could be done on the roof. How the heck were we going to pull this one off!? The only alternate space within the facility, the synagogue, had capacity for 40 people comfortably. We had 60 residents plus the staff that would assist them. How were we going to provide for privacy and care throughout the day? We could only think of the nightmare of trying to meet the expectations and needs of our large group; imagine the calling out, the screaming and demanding. This was going to be far from easy! We would certainly need *everyone's* cooperation to make this happen.

My greatest concern was for the residents with varying degrees of dementia, who comprised the vast majority of our group. How would they make sense of this? Such a disruption to their routine outside their familiar environment would escalate their confusion and exacerbate difficult and disruptive behaviors.

Rumors fly around a skilled facility; many residents knew about the evacuation before staff did. Some had already entered a panicked state, without remembering why. Since no one really had a clue as to what would be the best way to help such a diverse group of individuals deal with this, it seemed important to me to find out from the residents what *they thought* would most help them cope. After all, as a group, they had survived much, including multiple wars, a major depression, relocations, deaths of loved ones—nightmares in reality that were much worse than a temporary relocation. Surely they would have some clue about what could help them deal with stress, right? Maybe we should just ask them!

The social workers and recreational therapists went to these residents and met in groups and with individuals. In my meetings, the first words out of my mouth were "Thank you" for meeting with me and for helping to figure out the best way to go about this evacuation. I admitted that I didn't have a clue as to how to make this bearable for each resident, but I did have faith that they would be able to provide some insight for coping with this stressful situation. I sincerely needed their help.

Their reactions almost unanimously showed some degree of surprise that I was thanking them thinking that they had anything to offer that would help me. After all, I was the perceived expert. In all forums, however, I emphasized that while their ways of coping were perhaps different from mine, theirs were certainly successful—they were all still around, right? Our goal was to try to understand what helped get each individual get through the difficult times. Did a particular object—such as a soft afghan, or a picture, a stuffed animal or jewelry—provide them with a feeling of connection or comfort? Were there any particular foods or activities that felt nurturing to them? They came up with some very helpful thoughts and feedback for the group and for themselves. For some, the staff and family members helped to identify needs. Our exploration was fascinating and very helpful. We made our resident-specific and group-appropriate lists.

On the morning of the evacuation, we immediately thanked each person for helping us devise a plan. The thanking both acknowledged and reminded them that they helped to create the plan. When we were all convened in our tight space, we even had a discussion group about the topic of dealing with stress. Imagine getting 60 residents to talk about one topic! It took significant effort on the part of the entire team to keep us all focused and to get input from as many persons as possible but, once again, the residents were great. We talked about how they reacted to all of the "nerve-wracking experiences" they had survived throughout their many years. We talked about what helped to relieve stress and all the ways they have managed to "get through" the difficult times. Their group wisdom came from a total of over 4500 years of combined experience, which we drew together to create an article for their newspaper later that month. The article ended with this conclusion: "After reading this article, maybe the 'experts' will just come ask us, instead of spending all that money and time on researching" (JHA ⁊⁊, Fall, 1990).

The residents were great. None of anyone's worst fears came true. We made sure they received the credit they truly deserved throughout the day, both as a group and individually. We thanked them repeatedly, for we could not have done this without their help. We could clearly see the pride and accomplishment each of them experienced when we expressed thanks. It was extraordinary to me to experience the power of those words. Thanking them named their participation, their worth and their usefulness—particularly poignant with the institutionalized and the demented elderly, who all too often feel totally useless and worthless.

SUMMARY

During the course of her illness, the person with dementia becomes less able to participate in the world in familiar ways. She quickly learns that others see her as having no value—she feels that she has nothing to offer others, that she is no longer wanted. Her feelings of disconnection might even be intensified by our unwitting, well-intentioned efforts to protect her or ourselves from all the frustrations and disappointments that occur with her illness. We can easily do too much for her; we make decisions for her, direct her or assume that she is no longer capable of having any thoughts or feelings about the world around her. With all of our most open hearted and best of intentions, we might be missing what is possibly one of the most important things we can do for the person with dementia—receive her gifts.

Expressing thanks can be powerful evidence to the person with dementia that you received her unique personal contribution in connection. Offering a thank you lets the person know that both of you have been affected in similar ways and this strengthens your bond. Mr. Phillips and I both felt good about ourselves, because we were able to participate in helping the other person feel good. Lollie and I both were warmed by our mutual ability to connect because we engaged the other "important" person—I was important to her because she respected my professional title and education and she was important to me because I respected how much she gave to the world with profound consciousness. Kathryn and I felt good about ourselves because we effectively communicated with each other on various levels. And the evacuated residents and I both felt good about our usefulness—they were useful in helping to design a great plan and I was effective in helping to follow through with their plan to its successful completion.

There is mutuality in these connections. Each of us shares with the other as fully as possible. We both transform because the other entered the experience of the moment with us. In the expression of thanks, we move beyond our limited perspectives to acknowledge a mutual connection and its impact on both of us.

A simple thank you for something you received from *being with* the person who has dementia, brings the person back into the rhythm of human interaction and into feeling worthy, wanted, appreciated and useful. We both are energized and motivated to move forward, to continue our connection and to have more connections.

These sorts of interactions with persons with dementia have opened me over time to living in that peaceful, joyful and thankful place that Sara so clearly demonstrated. I find myself in a state of gratitude for the tools I've acquired from connecting with persons with dementia, for the role modeling I have received, for the many healing relationships—all of which move me into more gratitude in my everyday life.

It seems to come easily for me, having gratitude for something and thanking the person who has dementia. When I do have difficulty finding something to be thankful for, I pay attention to what surprises or delights me, or to whatever brings up joyful memories. It also helps to focus on the smallest things— an upturned corner of the mouth, an ever-so-slight squeeze of my hand or a long and comforting sigh during a peaceful moment. All of these confirm that we have met on common ground and I instantly fill with gratitude.

Being thankful about something when *being with* persons with dementia, however, is not simply about appreciation of the little things—even though that is a good place to begin if you are having trouble. As I hope every example throughout this book shows, persons with dementia are constantly surprising me with deep understanding about how to be in the world with consciousness and love, about how to adapt and cope with difficulties, about the value of being silent and living in the moment. These veritable pearls of wisdom have not been lost on me. They have brought on quantum shifts in my own learning and understanding. The big pearls might not come often in your relationships with persons who have dementia, but when they do, and you are open and ready to receive them, you will not be able to deny feeling thankful—and expressing your thank-you.

WORKING IT OUT

Feel thankful and practice the art of gratitude.

Transform Negative Perspectives

Look into your past and bring your attention to one specific event or situation that was extremely difficult or challenging for you. Now think of three things that you can be thankful for in relation to that challenging situation. Take some time with it. It doesn't matter how small your observations for thankfulness, but when you acknowledge their existence you create a shift—at least some of those negative feelings from the past will dissolve. It helps to broaden your view of the situation to include the wider picture. It helps to provide a more balanced perspective and to decrease the severity of the situation.

Repeat this exercise with other challenging events or situations in your life. With each shift and broadening of your perspective, you will increasingly be able to meet challenges with less fear and reticence. Hopefully, you will find comfort when you discover the positive aspects of your experience for which you can be thankful.

Thankfulness Pushups

MAKE A LIST

If you are a list-maker, list 25 things you appreciate that have happened to you today. Make the list at the end of each day. Now, don't panic! It will get easier each day you do it. It will certainly cultivate a focus on the good things in your life.

VISUALIZE THANKFULNESS

Look at each person you come into contact with and imagine that you are surrounding them with light, love and thanksgiving.

PRAY

Religious and wisdom traditions talk about the importance of spending some time each day in a sincere reflection on the gifts we have received in whatever ways they have manifested. Even if in a brief moment of time, the sincerity of the reflection will encourage the development of thankfulness.

RECALL HELPFUL PEOPLE

Settle into a cozy chair and let your mind open to the memories of a few people in your life who have been particularly helpful to you. Perhaps there was a person who encouraged you when you were growing up; perhaps someone gave you a gentle hug or a chocolate kiss that lifted your spirits. It doesn't have to be a person who changed your entire life—it could simply be a person who helped create a shift for you in a moment toward feeling better. Spend a few moments now with the memories of each person's helpfulness and the good feelings they helped draw out. Fill yourself with the gratitude from these precious moments and for these beautiful people having been a part of your life.

Keep a Thankfulness "Journal"

As you walk through the day, open your awareness to each person that you come in contact with. Pay attention to the details—what about that person brings a smile to your face; what about her manner has been helpful to you or raised your awareness; how has she made your day pass by more smoothly? See if there is something about her for which you can be actively thankful during your interactions with her.

Pay attention to the beauty around you—down to the little details. Notice the little things that can bring you joy and lead you to feeling thankful. No matter how small or large, write it down in your journal. At the end of the day, take a few moments to read through each entry and to reflect.

Commit to keeping this focus whenever you can—and do not judge yourself harshly for forgetting; try to let go of those gremlins. If a full day feels totally overwhelming and you know that it is just not going to happen, give yourself permission to *chunk it down* to size. In my earlier days of wanting to increase my awareness of feeling thankful, for example, the grocery store was my practice turf. I committed to truly paying attention to the persons I encountered in the grocery store as I picked up whatever was on my shopping list. It is amazing how a little personal interaction with a stranger can transform you both within an otherwise mundane experience. As I pushed the cart around, I noticed things that gave me joy and then made note of them, either by writing them down in a journal or holding the thought in my consciousness. Perhaps it was that wonderful store clerk who took time away from stocking shelves to personally escort me to the jars of sliced ginger. Perhaps it was seeing yet another three-year-old scream for the candy in the checkout line, sending me flashbacks of my boys when they were that age—how much more pleasant those candy-aisle moments are in hindsight! During my drive home, I would reflect and allow myself to fill with thankfulness. This exercise has successfully transformed grocery shopping from a drudge's task to an adventurer's playground, with endless possibilities and joys.

7 - Connections at the End of Life

If the dementing disease process cannot be reversed and the continuing deterioration cannot be changed, the person with dementia will eventually die. This might seem obvious, yet family members are frequently surprised when their loved one nears death. Even though they have become agile, adjusting to the changing demands of the disease over time, they freeze—hypnotized when death is imminent. One daughter, faced with the news of her mother's impending death said, "I never really believed she would actually die—she survived everything else all these years!"

So focused on the shifting needs of their loved one, some families put off thinking about the inevitable. When this happens, years of dementia can go by with family members silently fearing death and the strong emotions it unearths. Some consider death a failure—of the medical community to find a cure, of the person's will to live, of the family's ability to provide adequate attention and so on. With that sense of fear or failure comes a temporary paralysis that leaves family members stunned and helpless when death is actually at the door.

Thanks to the worldwide hospice movement, there is now a tremendous reserve of knowledge and help when it comes time to deal with dying. The hospice care movement has taught us how to respond to the needs of the dying person. As a result, family members and professionals have and show much more respect for the dying person's individuality and his unique end-of-life process. We know now that we are responsible to open to his particular needs, to help him resolve his specific concerns and to allow him full participation (to the degree he is able) in making decisions about his care. We are there to join him in his reflections as he tries to make sense of his life.

After years of experience as a medical social worker, however, I have found that the majority of people who accept this hospice practicum for being present, attentive and helpful at the end of a person's life do not understand how it all applies to end-of-life care for the person with dementia.

In 2003, I conducted an informal survey of 84 care professionals and family care providers on the ability of the person with dementia to participate in end-of-life care discussions or life reflections and review. Everybody agreed that it was important to remain open to the individual's needs throughout the progression of his disease. They stressed the importance of remaining available to help resolve the dying person's specific concerns, whether stated or evidenced.

Seventy-seven percent of my survey respondents, however, said that beyond the very early stage of the disease, the person with dementia was incapable of being included in decisions about his own end-of-life care, such as use of a feeding tube, IV, ventilator or planning for CPR and funeral arrangements. "They have no judgment anymore," was the common reason listed in the survey. Runner-up reasons included: "They can't put words together—how could I trust any decisions?" "They would only get upset," "It would only complicate things."

Ninety percent of the respondents thought that the person with dementia was incapable of processing at the end of life or of going through a life review at all. "How can they process when they can't put words or thoughts together," one person said, "or if they can't remember anything?" As a result of these kinds of blanket assumptions, many family members dread that their loved one who has dementia will not make peace with his God or die serenely because he will never come to terms with the events and actions of his life.

I ardently disagree with the global belief that the person with dementia is incapable of somehow participating in decisions and in end-of-life processing. In fact, I believe our traditional definitions, approaches and therapies need to stretch beyond the limits they have placed around the person with dementia.

I have experienced frequent opportunities during spontaneous islands of clarity with the person who has dementia to creatively explore his opinions and preferences regarding advance directives and decisions. I have witnessed and supported many persons—some with quite profound dementia—during a life review process in which they tried to make sense of their lives and their relationships with God and others. When we assume that the person with dementia cannot participate on these levels, we do him a great disservice.

The person with dementia who is near death is not immune to the issues that confront any other dying person. Actually, he continually has had to deal with these issues because of all the "little deaths" that occur along the path of his disease. Each day brings countless moments of his having to face another experience of loss: of his ability to be independent; to communicate and connect with others; and to process emotions and control his own thinking and basic physical functions. For the person with dementia, the final letting go of life comes after much practice of letting go throughout his decline. We can only imagine how constant is his challenge to maintain any semblance of self-esteem and personal dignity. When we participate in connection with him, we offer great support as he endures and processes all of his little deaths.

IF you are **LOST** as to how to support the person with dementia when his life is coming to an end, focus again on the basic principles discussed throughout this book. The end-of-life processes flow more smoothly as we effectively connect with the person who has dementia and participate in the rhythm of loving relatedness with him. Connecting with the person with dementia helps him advance through all of the "little deaths" of his decline and ease his eventual transition to death. It lets him continue to experience himself as a visible and worthy person.

My observations tell me that when a person with dementia is in a connected state with others, he has a greater potential for increased clarity, a greater potential for insights or "Aha!" moments, and a greater potential for connecting to levels of himself and the expanded field—the energy field that some call the "other side" or "heaven."

FIRST: GET COMFORTABLE
WITH YOURSELF

In order for a connection to happen between you and the person with dementia, it is up to you to try to reduce anxiety—yours as well as hers, since she will certainly pick up on your anxiety! An excellent antidote to anxiety about end-of-life care and death and dying is knowledge.

Learn about all the possible choices, the medications that are available and what other people have experienced. Talk with experts—geriatric specialists and hospice care professionals—about dignified, comfort-focused end-of-life care even if death is years away. They can provide a long-term view of the course of an illness, bring up considerations that need to be discussed early on and talk about ways the person can be made comfortable throughout her decline and into death.

By now, you might be hearing from your gremlins. There may be all sorts of little internal negative pop-up messages that will create barriers to being open to new information as well as to the person who needs your connection. If your gremlins are ever going to take stage, talking about death will most certainly be their cue.

When we know that someone is nearing death, our grief, fear, anger, anxiety—a full range of powerful feelings—can interfere with our best intention to connect with her. I have heard some family members and care providers say that only special people and saints are able to do this kind of work, implying that they themselves are not special and cannot deal with gremlins. If the wisdom principles **IF LOST** resonate with you, you *are* capable of being with the person who has dementia throughout her dying process. But first, it is very important to look within and check out whether you really want to participate—and if so, ask what might be in your way.

Sit in a relaxed position in a comfortable and quiet space and listen very carefully to the thoughts preventing you from an open, loving presence with the person who has dementia who is in her dying process. Focus once again on letting go of any of those barriers or old messages that create distance or blockage. At least try to send these gremlins and their disruptive messages on a little coffee break so that your full **I**ntention to connect can help you be present one moment to the next.

Next, revisit the need to **F**ree yourself of all of those opinions, judgments and assumptions that are sitting in the wings ready to take over as you see the person getting closer to death. Here is a common assumption, for example: there is a *Right* way to die—*the* universal process for everyone. It is this very assumption that leaves even those people who have a lot of experience with the dying at a sudden loss as to how to companion the person with dementia through the dying process. The person with dementia doesn't seem to follow the traditional and familiar—what some think of as *"Right"*—ways. Rarely. In my experience, the dying process of the person with dementia has been as unique and as unpredictable as the individual herself. This alone has been humbling and has made me very wary of my own assumptions!

MRS. JENKINS

Even at age 89 and with progressed dementia, Mrs. Jenkins was a proper and dignified lady, a true southern belle. Her hair was always just so, she moved with delicate grace and spoke gently to everyone. Well beyond the time that Mrs. Jenkins could no longer feed herself, she could still perfectly arch her little finger as she sipped afternoon tea and say, "Charming" with a distinct southern lilt. Unfortunately, her heart was having difficulty ridding her body of fluids. When medications and treatments were no longer effective, she went into congestive heart failure. Mrs. Jenkins was not going to be alive much longer.

I went into her room and sat by her bed. Holding her hand and simply being with Mrs. Jenkins had always been a calming joy for each of us. That particular afternoon, she was more alert than usual. She told me, amidst partial and incomplete wording, how Mr. Jenkins, whom I knew had died 32 years before, had come to see her. He told her about where they would travel next, she said, "so very far away." I told her that I would miss her, that I was happy for her and that I was grateful to her for everything she had meant to me over the past year. She said, "Oh, yes," then fell into silence.

After a while, she appeared worried and somewhat sad. I asked what was going on and she shook her head but said nothing. I remained with her, with touch, in calm and open presence. After about ten minutes, she very softly and rather apologetically said, "I have to go." The nurses had told me she could die at any time, and so it seemed that Mrs. Jenkins' time had come. I gave her a blessing and permission to go with Mr. Jenkins. She shook her head "No" and looked very sad but couldn't say anything. I told her that I would stay with her if she felt that would be helpful, and she nodded, yes.

As we sat together, I wondered what was keeping her here and so I occasionally asked her questions to explore what I assumed was her resistance. Perhaps she was having difficulty letting go of this world, so I said to her that sometimes it's very hard to leave everything and everyone you know and love. I thought that maybe there was some unfinished business that was pressing on her mind, so I asked her if there was anything she wanted me to tell her family or friends. Perhaps there was a concern about meeting her maker or facing judgment, so I empathized by saying that I could imagine it must be HUGE to think of finally meeting God face to face! I felt confident that I could help her through this; I had helped many others through their resistance to their final transitions from this life.

Mrs. Jenkins merely shook her head and shrugged at everything I said. Very gradually she began to look more frustrated and even sadder. She eventually said very softly, very discretely and with much embarrassment, "Pee." The poor woman! I was locked into my assumption that she was talking about the Big Going—her death—while she was just too lady-like to clearly state what she really needed. I sincerely apologized for not understanding her and quickly brought an aide to help her. About an hour later, with no further bumps along the way, Mrs. Jenkins smiled and very peacefully closed her eyes. Her heart and breathing stopped; her new journey began.

Immediately afterward, I had to work on letting go of my berating self-judgments over my mistake. The most important thing I learned was that I too readily assumed that Mrs. Jenkins feared dying, that she had difficulty leaving life or with resolving a life issue at the time of death. I didn't pause to observe the obvious or to reflect about the possibility that she might be one of those individuals who finds death a welcome relief from symptoms, or one who feels ready to move on. She loved life fully and appeared to be ready to go.

The dying and death of another may bring up fear, shock, sadness and rage about your own death. It is important to explore and accept such reactions—perhaps with the aid of an exercise at the end of this chapter. If you can accept your own pain reactions and emotional responses, you will be in a better position to accept the unique experiences of the person who is dying, to meet her on common ground and connect with her emotions. It is this connection that enables you to be compassionate throughout her processes. When you identify and lower your protective barriers, you will more fully open your heart and make yourself available to her experiences without resistance.

Death can be a very peaceful, grace-filled, joyous time—for the dying person as well as for those of us who accompany her toward her transition. The most helpful thing we can do is prepare ourselves to be as open and receptive as possible as the connections and her process unfolds. Our preparation includes an honest exploration of our gremlins, a letting go of our opinions and assumptions and a relaxing into the present moment with full attentiveness, inner silence and love. The goal is to be gentle with ourselves and with the person who has dementia. There is no need to force anything. As those moments in connection with the person who has dementia come and go, we can simultaneously open to the possibility that she may be able to express her preferences or to participate in decisions on some level. As those moments in connection happen, we can open to the possibility that she may be able to participate in end-of-life processing, perhaps in ways we do not fully understand.

PARTICIPATING IN DECISION-MAKING

Ideally, sometime early in the disease process, the person with dementia, as many family members as possible and other responsible parties talk over preferences and make conscious choices about end-of-life care. The first exercise at the end of this chapter can help you and your loved one begin this kind of discussion. Avoiding the dialogue only serves to magnify the uncertainties and burdens at the end of life.

HELEN

Helen was an amazing example of this ideal. The week following her diagnosis of Alzheimer's disease, she called together her three sons, two daughters, their spouses and the 12 grandchildren. She told me to bring my pen and paper to take notes because she said she wanted to make some decisions about how her life was going to play out. Helen said that the time may come when she will not be able to make decisions for herself and she asked me to present different possible scenarios of the future and to facilitate an open discussion. She wanted her family's input, understanding and consent.

She designated her first-born as her Health Care Agent to carry out her wishes should she become incapable of expressing her thoughts, and she wrote down her advance directive. The paperwork was signed on the spot—her next door neighbor came over to notarize all signatures. Helen stated her funeral preferences: "Please! No open casket!" she said emphatically. While everyone was still present, she even wrote her own obituary—"After all," she said, "I knew myself the best!" Each person was on board and her plan was to "sail through these choppy waters," taking in the loving support that surrounded her. They honored all of her wishes for the remainder of her life.

Unfortunately, countless people have faced the predicament of making decisions without ever having discussed preferences with their loved ones who have dementia. Many families found it too awkward or blatantly taboo to talk about the end of life. For others, there never seemed to be the right time, especially with a diagnosis of progressive dementia and no clear sense of a time frame for the decline to death. They might have been told that death could occur within a few years or stretch out over the course of ten or more years. If a vascular disease was involved, they heard death could come by a massive stroke within the next day or two, or that the person with dementia could inch along a gradual decline, as a result of the cumulative effects of several mini-strokes. The amorphous disease processes of persons with dementia seem to continually shift to thwart accurate predicting as to when death will occur.

Since death initially did not seem imminent to these family members, they expected that the moment to discuss such matters would clearly emerge at the appropriate time. Even more common was the hope that everything would take care of itself and they would not have to deal with the matter. Family members could shift focus to more pressing matters, such as managing the myriad details of their loved one's moment-to-moment existence. As a result, it did seem sudden then, when the person with dementia was not able to talk about it any more and someone had to step up and make decisions.

When to allow treatment or not, and when to accept or not, that the disease is continuing its course, become dramatically complicated decisions when the person has dementia. The effects of the variety of medical interventions on the person with dementia can be so individual that it is difficult to predict its impact beforehand. For example, the person may have another acute condition, a tumor in the colon or the lung for instance, and a surgical procedure is offered. Will general anesthesia increase his confusion permanently or will he eventually go back to his baseline—pre-surgical—level of confusion? Will he be able to tolerate or participate in post-surgical rehabilitation with his level of confusion? If the consideration is for a feeding tube, oxygen, IV therapies or medications, will he experience increased comfort or will he be frightened by these foreign pieces of equipment attached to his body? When he can't understand or remember what is causing the pain or why it is there, can the right balance be found between decreasing his anxiety about the pain while not increasing his confusion?

The family becomes very conflicted too—they will have to live with the consequences of their decisions. The decision-making becomes overwhelming. So, the family often turns to friends or others who might consider themselves experts. This often adds to rather than relieves an already emotionally charged burden. One so-called expert often has a compelling argument for one option which directly opposes the advice of another friend-expert. Each expert backs up his own opinions with strong ethical beliefs, such as the right to a dignified death, what constitutes "dignified" or even God's will. Frustration and confusion snowballs because the advice is based in the personal preferences, judgments and prejudices the advice-giver genuinely believes—that his own global reality is the way things are and how it is done. Period.

To me, any sweeping generalities, any *this is just the way it is* regarding end-of-life care, sends up a big, red flag and becomes eminent cause for hesitation. No categorically Right or Wrong intervention exists (though I'd love it if it did!). By intervention, I mean any course of action that will affect the person's treatment.

Each intervention is full of possible decisions that can best be made after family members study the full spectrum of choices available. After considering the unique needs of the individual and after amassing as much medical information as possible, then family members can begin to consider an intelligent and compassionate decision. I say 'consider' because there is one other person, the person with dementia, who I strongly advocate be included in the discussion before finalizing any life-and-death choices.

There's the rub—how can the person with dementia be included if he is not able to clearly respond to questions regarding his preferences? Unfortunately, it has been the norm to rule out including the person with dementia way too early in the disease process. More to the point, my experience teaches me that it is very important to discuss medical condition and decision-making while the person with dementia is in the room—whether or not we think he can understand; whether or not he is able to indicate a conscious awareness of the discussion. His potential to participate is possible; it does exist—a moment of clarity can occur or a family member might see or hear him express an opinion.

ROBERT

Robert told me he was stalwart to the bone the first day I met him. A navy man, he knew the right way, which was his way, to do everything. His daughter, Liz, worked very hard to support his living independently in his home of 65 years. It was quite the tough balancing act for her as each day of the six years after his diagnosis of Alzheimer's presented new challenges. She took steps to assure herself that he was safe amidst his mounting confusion, and discovered creative ways to help him to experience that he was handling life on his own. However, the day she feared most finally came: the family home burned to the ground. "Thank God I showed up when I did!" she said. "At least I could get him out of the house or I would have lost him, too! I can't figure out how he kept getting more cigars. I took them away a thousand times over the years." That was the week Robert came to live in the facility.

Four years later, Robert was no longer taking in enough nutrition to stay alive. His dementia might have progressed to the point that the signals from his brain were not effective enough for him to know what to do with whatever was in his mouth. He squirreled the food and occasionally some food and fluids would trickle down his throat. At times this triggered his swallowing a bit of something but mostly he just choked on it. It appeared that his lungs began to fill with whatever wasn't properly swallowed and pneumonia developed. Or, perhaps it wasn't aspiration pneumonia; maybe he wasn't eating well because he was initially weakened by the pneumonia. The physician needed to have a very direct discussion with Liz to know how to proceed medically, since there was no advance directive on Robert's chart. Liz told us that she had learned long ago not to make any decisions for her father so she wanted to have the discussion in Robert's room, "…just in case he can somehow let us know," she guessed. It didn't feel rational to her, but she felt it was important.

When the physician, Liz and I walked into Robert's room, he was in his recliner chair with eyes closed. This recent change in Robert's ability to eat was accompanied by a more vacant appearance. If he opened his eyes at all, he stared off in the distance, expressionless. He hadn't spoken in months, but he was receptive to calming touch and vocal qualities and could respond to visitors with deep sighs of relief and comfort. At our greeting, Robert took a long, deep breath but did not open his eyes or respond in any other way.

The physician introduced the reason for our being there—that we all cared deeply for Robert and that we wanted to discuss his change in condition and to talk about some choices that we might consider. In a wonderfully caring and patient way, the physician laid out Robert's scenario and described all the possible interventions in reference to his recent change in condition. Liz held her father's hand the entire time to give him a physical sign that he was a part of the discussion; she did not want him to feel that everyone was talking over and around him.

Liz said she knew about her father's past decisions to have IVs used in his care, and she felt he would want IV antibiotics now to address his acute condition, the pneumonia. She said that if the decline from the pneumonia was causing his swallowing problem, then dealing with that might make him more comfortable for a longer period of time and possibly get him back to eating better. So, she easily voted to provide him with IV antibiotics. During the entire discussion up to this point, there had been no response from Robert. Even when his daughter asked him directly, he remained very still.

Liz continued saying that in her heart she felt that the IV choice might be just a temporary fix—that the pneumonia would most likely reappear if her father's inability to take in adequate nutrition and fluids was due to the progression of his Alzheimer's disease, and not pneumonia. The physician then talked about the possibility of placing a G-tube if Robert's ineffective swallowing was a permanent condition of his disease. This small plastic tube could be surgically inserted into the stomach and would allow him to take in nutrition while bypassing the need to chew and swallow. The doctor outlined the pros and the cons and the potential risks and rewards of this decision. Suddenly, Robert began rocking back and forth in his chair, his brow furrowed, his eyes open and his rate of breathing twice what it had been. We had to ask ourselves, why now? Why was he agitated at that moment? He certainly wasn't able to tell us with words what was going on for him, but we suspected that he was responding to the feeding-tube discussion.

We spent the whole afternoon checking and double-checking Robert's reactions, as we approached the topics from various angles. The physician, Liz and I each separately discussed with Robert the placing of an IV antibiotic and G-tube among other topics, both alone with Robert and with groupings of different people in his room. The only times Robert consistently showed agitated reactions were those when we mentioned placement of a G-tube. By day's end, we were convinced that he was quite clearly making his wishes known, even though our rational minds did not ever dream this would have been possible considering his level of confusion. When Liz told him that we would not talk any more about it and that the G-tube would not be inserted, Robert breathed that familiar long, deep and comforting sigh. We honored what we all knew was his wish.

I would much rather err on the side of assuming that the person with dementia *can* participate in his decisions about end-of-life care, rather than assuming he can't. It happens more than one would expect that during an open discussion, the person with dementia pops into a particular moment of clarity and clearly provides input. Like Robert, he is able to communicate his stance in consistent, nonverbal ways. Perhaps it is an opportunity to allow him to absorb whatever information he can about his condition, on whatever levels he may be capable of hearing and understanding. His presence during the discussions provides the opportunity for the potential of his participation and understanding.

In some families, the person with dementia becomes agitated when anyone brings up the illness or end-of-life decisions. Maggie lived in fear of jinxing her condition by talking about such things. Any mention of death or her illness upset her even in the very last weeks of her long decline. We certainly honored her need and talked privately with her family about necessary decisions.

In other families, the children are the ones who have difficulty talking about life and death in their parent's presence. In these situations, it is often the family member's emotional response to hearing about end-of-life care choices that the person with dementia picks up on and reflects back. It is important for everyone to remember that each person comes to these discussions with his own unique perspectives, opinions and emotional buttons that can dramatically complicate any consensus for action. It might be necessary to call in a medical social worker and a spiritual counselor, to help sort out concerns of both the person with dementia and the family as the need to make choices arises. Also, many facilities have highly active, multidisciplinary ethics committees that can help physicians, patients and families walk through the at times highly complicated decision-making process and come to a resolution.

MRS. BARBER

Another way to include the person with dementia who cannot participate in the moment is to talk to as many people as possible—her family members, friends and associates—about past events or conversations that might reveal her perspective—what she would do or decide. Many persons, either before diagnosis or well into the disease process, can be reluctant to enter into emotionally charged end-of-life concerns directly with immediate family, but will open up with a close friend or a care provider. Being a good detective and asking around can prove to be highly enlightening. Mrs. Barber's neighbor, for example, very clearly remembered a day several years before when she and Mrs. Barber were watching a news program about a woman who was being kept alive by tubes and machines. The neighbor recalled how angry Mrs. Barber became, saying, "NOT ME! I'll never let them do ANY of that to ME!" This was good information for Mrs. Barber's niece, the responsible party in this case. It told her how her aunt felt, at one point in her life. This added to the niece's much-needed resources for making a decision that would be best for her aunt in the current time frame.

COMING TO PEACE WITH THIS LIFE

Robert N. Butler, a groundbreaking geriatric psychiatrist, has written for decades about the importance of a life review for people who are nearing death. In an article written for the *Journal of American Geriatric Society*, he states that we go through a process of progressively remembering more of our past experiences. Our unresolved conflicts tend to surface for reexamination and integration. This life review process can help us find new meaning and significance to our life and help to reduce fear and anxiety about death. It is a practice that helps prepare us for death by satisfying our drive to put our lives in order.

Counselors, therapists and social workers have done extraordinary work helping people make peaceful closure at the end of life. Most of these same workers, however, have difficulty seeing the relevance of this work with persons who have dementia. After all, they think someone who is no longer capable of processing information in familiar ways cannot gain awareness. And even if she could, the gains from one visit most certainly would be lost by the next visit.

I, on the other hand, assert that to assume the person with

dementia is not capable of looking at her life at all is to gravely underestimate not only her potential but the power of what appears to be a natural instinct to make peace with a life lived.

Her thought processes and access to logical thinking certainly change with the progression of dementia, but we cannot assume that they never occur or are not possible. Each day can be filled with moments of reliving her past because her past is often being experienced as her present day world. Who is to say that she is not attempting, on some level, to find the meaning or significance of that period of time? Who is to say some unresolved conflict is not resurfacing for reexamination and hopeful reintegration?

She might be dealing with the emotional content of events in a way that is different from what we would normally perceive to be traditional therapeutic processing at the end of life. We also may never really know fully how her processing plays out, or is resolved. I would still like to encourage everyone to open to the possibility that persons with dementia can indeed experience end-of-life review and processing.

MRS. SANDOVAL

I made an appointment to talk with Mrs. Sandoval's daughter, Fran, before I met the woman herself, our most recent addition to hospice care. Mrs. Sandoval was 99 years old when she came to us because of end-stage liver disease, complicated by dementia that resulted from a series of strokes she had suffered over the years.

Fran said that her mother's dementia had progressed to the point where she spoke mostly in her native Armenian tongue, even though she had had few opportunities to speak the language since the age of eight. She said her mother had survived extreme poverty and hardship, multiple wars, horrid physical abuse and the eradication of her entire family. "In whatever language," Fran said, "she hasn't made much sense in the past six months…but oh, can she still love!"

I knocked on the door to announce that I was entering her room. Mrs. Sandoval was in bed and looked at me with a frown, trying to identify me. As I approached her, her face rapidly changed into delight. She reached out to take both of my hands and asked with a heavy accent, "Who are you?" I introduced myself and told her I was her hospice social worker but she laughed and said, "No, no. I know who you are! You are an angel!" She kept shaking my hands with the delight and surprise of a child and gazed at me with laughing, loving eyes. Every three minutes, Mrs. Sandoval asked who I was. Again and again we repeated the same dialogue, with her saying, "No, you are an angel" followed by our joyous exchange until finally after a long pause she said, "…or you're Mrs. Sugarman's daughter." That made us both laugh uproariously and we spent the rest of our visit in that joyous connection.

During the second visit, however, Mrs. Sandoval was in a very different place. She was watching an animal show on television—two alligators were competing for dominance. When I greeted her, she just kept staring at the television saying, "Such fighting. Such fighting. I don't understand. Such fighting in this world." I was not able to distract her with any of my exploratory questions; all of her energy was consumed by her own thoughts. Even after we turned the television off, she repeated her statements about the fighting in this world. Mrs. Sandoval held onto my hands and looked worried and confused, as she appeared to try to find the answer or reason.

I told Mrs. Sandoval that I, too, didn't understand why there has been so much fighting and pain in this world. I let the questioning go and sat with her, in love and silence. After about 20 minutes, she looked up and let out a sighing, "Ahhhhhhh." The light bulb clearly went on above her head. For the rest of the visit, she smiled and kept repeating the phrase, "The Mountain can't handle the pain. The Mountain can't handle the pain." I asked her to explain what this meant and she just kept repeating the phrase. Whatever it meant, it was clearly the answer she was seeking. So, we shared hugs and the joy that she had found her answer. At the end of our visit, we thanked each other and I told her I would return in a few days.

The next day, the facility called and told me that Mrs. Sandoval was actively dying, that it seemed she had only a few hours left. Fran was already with her mother when I arrived. Mrs. Sandoval was very peaceful as we sat by her bedside. Fran talked about her mother as a beautiful woman who had given exquisite gifts of wisdom to everyone throughout her life. I asked Fran about the expression "The Mountain can't handle the pain" and she smiled while recalling a folk tale from Armenia:

There was a time when the people of the world would climb up the mountain and deposit their pain onto the mountaintop. They would then be able to return to their villages, happy and content. There was no fighting, no war in this land.

But then the day came when the people climbed up the mountain to deposit their pain and the mountain said to them, "I cannot handle the pain." The people were forced to walk down the mountain and to hold onto their pain.

Fran explained that the tale was told to her mother as a child to help explain the reason for war, poverty, famine and pain in the world. Mrs. Sandoval's recollection of this folk tale the day before helped to create an emotional shift that suddenly allowed everything to make sense to her. She was not able to verbally share with me the process she went through, but she clearly came to some form of resolution of what was upsetting her in that moment. Her anxiety and confusion over the fighting in the world were released. Perhaps a part of her process was to resolve questions about her God and how such fighting in the world could coexist with Mrs. Sandoval's loving God. Perhaps her life took on a different meaning and her God made more sense. Whatever her process, she very openly and lovingly welcomed death, closing her eyes for the last time, with her daughter and me by her side, each of us holding her hands.

DEBORAH

It appeared as though the past was haunting Deborah. As her dementia progressed, she gradually lost her old entrenched abilities to hide her emotions. Particularly during our time together, she could no longer divert her attention from horrible, resurfacing memories of her mother and all the verbal and physical abuse she suffered. Amidst what to me were nonsensical words and statements, she revealed snippets of her past—she was just seven years old and was supposed to give her little brother, Seth, a bath to help her mother one evening. She didn't know he couldn't sit up on his own or that he couldn't keep his head above the water; how rapidly he drowned! Deborah's punishment went on well after her mother's death as she continued the lineage of emotional distancing and verbal abuse toward her only child, a son she named Seth.

Seth was an extraordinarily loving man. He was proud to say, "I stand before you, a product of years of therapy costing thousands of dollars and eventually finding forgiveness through God!" He had great compassion for his mother's pain. He told me how his mother insisted on bringing a doll with her the day she moved into the facility but, as his mother became more confused, she was increasingly fearful of the doll. She would not let anyone take her baby out of the room, but she could not bear to look at it either and asked someone to place him on the top shelf of the closet.

Each time Seth or I came to visit, Deborah motioned to us to open the closet door so we could see that her baby was safe. Over time, she became more fearful when we opened the closet door; she was afraid to leave the baby there, afraid to have us take it out and afraid to hold him herself. Once the closet door was closed and we reassured her that the baby was safe, Deborah eventually calmed down and enjoyed a loving interaction with us, "these nice strangers", as she called us, having lost her ability to identify our relation to her.

One day, I greeted Deborah who once again pointed fearfully at the closet asking me open to it. That day, however, she repeatedly said, "Bad mommy," while hitting herself on the arm. I asked, "Who, Deborah?" An anguished "ME!" was her response. Deborah appeared to be having increasing difficulty stuffing down her bad-mommy negative tapes, could not move beyond them and seemed to be struggling for some resolution.

Here was my dilemma. To try to help her analyze and to sort out the connections from her past would not be possible, particularly considering her dementia. I also agree with Edwin Schneidman, author of *Death: Current Perspectives*, whose opinion is that no one has to die in a state of psychoanalytic grace. So how could I help Deborah to at least achieve some psychological and emotional comfort in her present moments so she could move forward and out of this painful place?

I figured that the only way to connect with her was to meet her where she was in her past and talk with her as she perceived herself, a new mother who didn't know how to be a good one. I closed the closet door and went over to hug her, saying repeatedly as we rocked together, "All mommies need help knowing how to be a mommy, Deborah." I eventually asked her if she wanted me to teach her how to be a good mommy and she excitedly said, "Oh, yes!"

And so we began our process. On each of my visits, I walked into Deborah's room and reminded her that she told me she wanted the Mommy Classes. Initially, she remained fearful of letting me take the doll out of the closet. So, for a few visits, I would go over to the closet and talk with the doll, make silly faces and hold its hand playfully. Deborah became curious about her baby's responses and she soon let me take the doll out of the closet, hold it and talk lovingly to it. After about three visits, she let me show her how to take care of the doll— comb its hair, sponge bathe it and change its clothes.

At each visit, I reviewed what she had learned from previous visits and I told her how well she did—the memory cues were extremely important to give her a sense of process and progress. Very gradually, Deborah was able to hold her baby by herself and to provide care with confidence. After two months, she proudly called herself a good mommy and showed her baby to every passer-by. Her baby never left her side for the remaining five months of her life.

What about her son, Seth? He called the doll his new brother and continued to visit every day after work and to share his mother's joyful interactions with her baby and him. Three days before Deborah's death, she had a particularly clear evening. She turned to Seth, pulled his hand to her face and said, "You know, my dear, I love you very much." Seth told me this was the first time in his life that his mother ever said those words to him.

Sometimes a person with dementia, like Deborah, lives her present moments as though she were back in a problematic time of her life—reliving events or situations that were and consequently are now upsetting. Because of the dementia, she can no longer stuff down emotions, divert attentions or cover up upsetting and distasteful events and reactions. When we can enter her world, which is often in the past, and remain available as a loving presence, we have the opportunity to escort her along a process that will lead her into a more peaceful place. I must admit that it was not every week that I saw a person show such clear processing as Deborah entered. Some persons with dementia appear to "work it out" internally, in very private ways. For some others, the difficult moment and memory seem to be forgotten as she shifts into the next moment, perhaps into another time frame and a different memory. But I maintain that the possibility for the person with dementia to experience positive change is maximized when she is in the rhythm of a loving connection.

Life Review as Spiritual Inventory

An important part of any person's end-of-life processing is the looking back through life to discover any meaning or significance to her having been on earth. Enid Schwartz, in an excellent seminar entitled *Understanding and Effectively Managing End-of-Life Issues*, emphasizes the importance of including a kind of spiritual inventory as part of this life review:

How have I used the gift of human life? What have I learned about tenderness, love, vulnerability, communion, courage, strength, power and faith? What am I thankful for, what has been most important to me? What have I learned from interactions with others and how have I coped with life's tragedies? What has helped most to open my heart to being able to experience the presence of Spirit? What have been my gifts to the world that have made it perhaps just a little better than when I entered it?

As a person reviews her life, she has the opportunity to look for pieces of information that might help her discover her own personal truths, which then can lead her to understand what her life has been about. Her life review leads to what has really mattered; she then can accept her life and let it go. As Stephen Levine, author of *Healing into Life and Death*, states, "we can't let go of anything we do not fully accept."

The person with dementia, even one who is well into the disease process, can often be easily drawn into a life review. One such person might not be able to remember who you are or what she just had for lunch, but she can astound you with details about her earlier years. She might even be experiencing that earlier time frame in the present moment.

Unfortunately, we tend not to think of these things as strengths or assets that can support her life review. Most often we think that the person with dementia has decreased ability to conceptualize as the disease progresses, and even quite early in the disease, her ability to extract bits of information, piece them together and understand the significance of her life, is beyond her reach.

Here, however, is where you can be extremely effective in helping the person with dementia throughout the entire process of her decline. You can encourage the sharing of her life story, listen with a nonjudgmental and open heart, and help reflect back to her what most stands out to you as a unique gift she brought to the world, something that she will be leaving behind, something that has made it a better place.

Even as the person is actively dying and does not appear to be participating with this world in any discernible ways, it is very important to find opportunities to review her life and to offer reflections. Family members are an essential part of this process. In my hospice work, a major part of my responsibility is to be with family members and to help them through their own grieving process as their loved one approaches death. At times, I would not get the chance to meet the family or the person with dementia until she was in her last minutes to hours of life. What became an effective function was for me to be available to the family while being in the room with the dying person who had dementia, and to simply ask questions about who this person has been throughout her life.

THE WHEELERS

I got a call from our nurse during my early weeks as a hospice social worker. She asked me to go to an extended care facility to meet with the Wheeler family. Even though Fannie Wheeler's Alzheimer's disease had progressed for

11 years and she had not been eating anything substantial for over two months, her family members could not agree to make the decision to bring in additional hospice services. Two daughters were certain that hospice was only for people with cancer; a son and his three children never really believed Fannie was going to die; and another son was certain that hospice caregivers would merely give up on his mother, maybe drug her to death and have her die before her time. Only one daughter and her four children thought that hospice care would help. They finally all agreed to meet with our hospice nurse who cleared up all of these misconceptions and helped them understand our function to provide comfort care on multiple levels.

Although the family finally agreed to bring in hospice care, the timing felt unfortunate to me. Fannie, by this point, was in her last moments of life—not a lot of time, I thought, for Fannie and her large, diverse family to find some peace with the ending of her life.

I was wrong.

When I entered the room, all five children and seven grandchildren were standing like islands of sadness around Fannie's bed—all so painfully reluctant to let this woman's life end, yet not knowing how to be with each other or Fannie. Fannie was not responsive but appeared to be at ease and comfortable. They asked me questions about some of the physical symptoms that might manifest as Fannie let go of life. Answering them gave me an opportunity to normalize the dying process, to provide them all with a comforting presence and to role model how to be with Fannie. Suddenly, one of her sons drew the line, saying, "You better not come in here like the others. I am NOT going to tell my mother it is okay for her to die!!!"

I told him that of course it was not okay for him that his mother was dying! He loved her very much, he didn't want her to die, and he didn't want her to get the impression that he no longer cared, and that is exactly what saying okay could mean to her. This is one of the misconceptions about making closure with the person who is dying. Giving permission is often understood to mean that if I say okay, I am pressing the button or pulling the switch that sends my loved one over to the other side. Giving permission cannot control the matter. What is important, however, is to help the dying person with dementia to understand, on whatever levels she is capable, that the lives of those she cares about will go on, albeit with grieving, that she made an impression and had an impact in the world while she was here. With our gentle, compassionate touch and our loving connection, we can let her know her impact on us and we can say good-bye sometimes even without words.

Since I knew absolutely nothing about Fannie, I began asking the Wheeler family what she had been like. Over the next hours, the family revealed several chapters of Fannie's life. There were the basic how-when-and-where of her life, the number of people in her family of origin, significant births and deaths. I learned that her parents died young and that she took the three youngest siblings and made sure they were raised well and had a college education. After putting all of her own children through college, she went back to get her GED and then went to college herself.

"You know she was 74 when she got her bachelor's degree?"

"She was so proud!" "We were all so proud of her! She is an amazing woman!" Gradually more family stories emerged.

"Remember the time Grammy chased Gramps around the house with a wooden spoon the day she finally caught him putting liquor in the fruit cake."

"So THAT was the secret to her fruit cake! You just gotta love her spunk, don't you?"

"Then there was the time she saw me toss a gum wrapper on the ground and made me clean up all the trash on the ground at Flat Creek Park every Sunday for two months!"

"Boy! You make her sound like a tyrant!"

"Not at all! She taught me right from wrong. Why do you think I'm a cop?"

"Or, how she used to always mail a little care package to us when we were away from home with a note that said something like, 'Just so you know you are always a part of me.'"

"Man, I hope she knows how much she will always be a part of us!" Bob reflected sadly.

"She does," I could honestly say. "You just told her so."

Within the next few moments, Fanny very peacefully took her last breaths.

Fannie's children and grandchildren gracefully went beyond their pain and isolated grieving into communal sharing of the joys, disappointments, laughter, tears, wisdom, strength, love and support that Fannie gave to all of them. She led a good life and each of them could talk about how they were better for having such a beautiful role model in their lives.

Fannie was there to experience it all on whatever levels she could. We may not have seen evidence of her taking in what was being said, but each person with dementia, as we have heard about persons in a comatose state, has the potential of hearing and experiencing everything in her environment. Perhaps her heart resonated with the love and gratitude of those who were speaking in the room. Perhaps as she wavered in the realm between life and death, she was able to hear clearly what she could not take in fully, while still in her physically limited body. Even if Fannie could only take in a fraction of what was said or felt, it was an extraordinary gift to let her know how vital she was to those whose lives she touched. It could have been exactly what she needed to allow her to fully accept her life and to let go with an open spirit.

Of course, some family stories are much less colorful and are in fact very dark. Sometimes there is a raging alcoholic, abusive narcissist, sexual offender or irresponsible abandoner who leaves a lot of pain and disruption in her wake. Sometimes telling a parent's life story helps bring a damaged son or daughter to insight about how their mother was a product of a horrible childhood herself. At times the only good this person did was to make her child's life possible, or bestow gifts on the rest of the world, not her own family. Talking with friends, care providers and companions to get a broader picture of this person's lifetime can expand perspectives and be very helpful.

Life Review and the Role of Religion

If the person with dementia has ever followed a religious tradition, I urge that a cleric or a spiritual counselor participate in his end-of-life processing. Even if the person with dementia has not been to religious services since childhood, he still often goes back to those early roots when he perceives himself as being in that earlier time frame. He may need to hear that he will be cared for when he dies. He may benefit from the blessings and the comfort that a religious figure can provide with traditional rituals and prayers, readings and simply being present in the room. It is amazing how the power of the cloth can help ease his transition, whether or not we think he is aware.

Ideally, this religious figure not only provides comfort through prayer but also communicates effectively and listens to the needs of the person with dementia and to those of the family members. Hopefully, he or she is willing and able to assist in a spiritual inventory and to tackle some of the more difficult questions about life, death and God. These explorations, again, can be directly with the person who has dementia or in his presence via discussions with others in the room. If it is very clear that the person with dementia would not want clergy present, hospice can provide extraordinary spiritual counselors, who can be of great assistance in the end-of-life spiritual process.

OPENING TO THE EXPANDED FIELD

It is amazingly common that a person who is near death talks about or shows that she is having spiritual experiences that you might not be able to share or understand. These experiences do not necessarily mean that death is imminent; they can occur months or even years before the person actually makes the transition into death. Most of us have heard stories about how persons near death have seen a bright white light or have interacted with loved ones who have already died. Sometimes, the person who is dying has said she hears "music of the spheres" or feels the sensation of "a comforting, big hug of an angel." Each person's experience is unique and is reported by persons of all races, economic groups, religions, ages, genders...and all levels of cognition.

Are these experiences real? Among those of us who are not close to dying, the question raises a debate full of strong opinions. Some say that chemical changes in one's body near the end of life probably act as a hallucinatory agent. Others believe that what I call the expanded field of energy and others might call heaven, the other side or the spirit world, initiates these experiences. To me, finding proof and cause does not matter.

To the dying person, the experiences are very real and from my observations they almost universally allow the person, with or without dementia, to die in great comfort and peace. The transition into death frequently becomes more user-friendly and less overwhelming or scary when the person sees what she most often perceives as life beyond this world.

GINGER

I went to Ginger's home to meet with her family who were having a really tough time, I was told. It was no wonder. Ginger had been living quite happily with her husband, two adult daughters, a son-in-law and three grandchildren in a two-story home in the suburbs. Four weeks prior to my visit, she fell down a flight of stairs and hospital tests revealed a rapidly growing cancerous brain tumor. According to her physician, Ginger probably had one or two months to live. Two weeks later, the family brought Ginger home, placed her in bed on the first floor, and called hospice to ask what to do next.

The family said they needed to meet with me first, because they didn't want Ginger to hear their insecurity and craziness, as they called it. We talked about the logistics of hospice services and I fielded questions which helped them vent many of their fears and concerns. Along the way, I discovered quite a bit about this woman whom they all held in such high regard. They described her as the most loving person on the face of the earth. She totally enjoyed her life, particularly her time spent with her family and "MANY" friends, her traveling the world, her pets—and all animals, for that matter—and being in the garden with her flowers. Ginger loved life so unabashedly that she was not planning on dying—ever. "It's just plain too much fun being around here," she had said more than once. "Why would I leave this...for nothing?"

So now, Ginger's family did not know what to make of the fact that she really was going to die. Her husband was very concerned about whether or not she could go to heaven (his personal belief system) if she didn't believe in one, which she did not. Their best hope at this point they thought was that death would be quick and painless.

We all then went into the room so I could meet Ginger. To my surprise, she was in a hospital bed in a very poorly lit and stark room. There were no pictures or decorations and only one folding chair in the far corner. Other than that, there were her oxygen tank and some hospital supplies. She was basically in a large coffin already—it was really quite eerie.

I pulled the chair over to her bedside, sat down to be at eye level with her and touched her hand while introducing myself. She firmly held onto my hand and stared at me with very little expression. Ginger had not been able to speak since leaving the hospital. Her physician's best guess was that the tumor had already destroyed the speech center of the brain. I asked the family if they had to renovate the room to make space for Ginger, trying to see if the starkness was deliberately created. It had been. Her husband said that they thought it might be easier for Ginger to let go of life if the things she loves aren't around her; so they removed everything. Even their dog and cats were banned from the room.

As Ginger kept holding my hand, I gave them all examples of other person's experiences as each approached the end of life. I said that the letting go is a process that does not seem to mean putting aside all of what life held but rather acknowledging the life lived and honoring its multifaceted beauty, discoveries, teachings and gifts. A part of the letting go is opening to the possibility that love exists beyond death—even if only in the hearts of those who have been touched by that person's love. Another aspect of the letting go process is often found with the opening of that person's heart to thankfulness, love and the possibility that something might exist beyond death. I told Ginger and her family that surrounding her with all she has so passionately loved could help her remain open and loving for both the time left to her and in her transition into death.

This beautiful family flew with my suggestion! I returned the following week to a brightly lit room filled with fresh flowers and plants, travel posters, pictures, places for people to sit and to hang out in comfort. There were animals jumping on and off her bed; the room was full of life! What was more extraordinary was Ginger's expression as she looked at everyone and everything in the room— that ear to ear grin her family recognized.

Her husband told me about an incident that happened two nights before my second visit. He was sitting by the side of her bed and noticed she was looking at something right next to him. "She was in awe," he said. "She kept reaching to touch whatever it was and looking at me too to see if I could see it, but I saw nothing. Then she very weakly said something almost inaudible—'Angel'—and her eyes welled up with tears, as she looked totally bathed with love." He said that she had not stopped smiling since that moment and he strongly felt that she had the evidence she needed that there is a heaven. Whether or not this was Ginger's specific reality, she clearly experienced something that increased her comfort, love and peace for the remaining weeks of her life.

Sometimes when the person with dementia sees spirits or angels that others do not see, she becomes noticeably uncomfortable. If her images or experiences are upsetting her, it is important to check out why. The upsets might be due to a systemic physiological change, which can bring on nightmare-like hallucinations or delusions. In this case, an appropriate dosage of prescribed medication can correct the imbalance so the upsetting visions don't recur. In another scenario, disturbing images indicate an adverse reaction to medication(s). From my experience, however, the most common cause for the person's discomfort when she sees presences in the room is that she thinks she is going crazy or she is worried that others think she is going crazy. In these cases, our ability to normalize her experience of spirit presences provides all the comfort she needs to open to the love that is surrounding her.

MISS ANDERSON'S SPIRIT

The one person I can remember who had a particularly unique concern about a presence was Miss Anderson. To the people she met throughout her life, she had always described herself as a schoolmarm. "I never married but I am the mother of thousands," she was proud to say. She had become far more confused and forgetful over the years but was aware enough to know that her body was "about to kick it off."

One morning, she looked very concerned and motioned me over to her bedside. She asked if I saw the little boy standing at the bottom of the bed. I said that I didn't see him and asked her to describe him to me. "He has red hair, checkered pants and green suspenders," she said, "pleasant enough, I suppose, but why is he there?" I asked Miss Anderson if she could ask the little boy that question and she quickly responded, "Oh, no! We haven't been properly introduced." I suggested that this might be just one of those rules she lived by over the years that she could relax just a little. Maybe just this one time she could consider introducing herself to him, since she was the only one who could talk with this little boy in the moment. "Well, I'll have to just think about that," she said.

The next morning, her aide called me to the unit, saying she was concerned that "Miss Anderson has lost it!" She told me how she walked into Miss Anderson's room that morning and heard her talking to thin air, saying, "How do you do. My name is Miss Anderson. How do you do. My name is Miss Anderson." I laughed, and told her about the day before. Miss Anderson had clearly decided to introduce herself to her new little friend—the one whom she would eventually call her little precious one who would help her, as she said, "...feel at home with God."

This is an expansion on the more traditional discussions of the value of time spent with the person who has dementia. I have come to understand that my positive, nonjudgmental, open, loving connection with the person who has dementia mirrors the experience many persons with or without dementia have as each opens to the 'other side' at the end of life. Just as loving connected relationships in her day-to-day world help the person with dementia remain open to being with others in this world, so it appears that our loving connectedness may free her to connect with loving presences that appear to her, but not to us. At minimum, the person is more willing to share her experiences with those of us who can provide opportunities for a loving connection. By being with her in connection, we encourage a gentle balance that will create less conflict and will ease her eventual transition. Connecting with her in her world, puts us in a better position to offer support along her sometimes bumpy path.

Processing 'Between Worlds'

There are times when I see or feel that a person with dementia is stuck between this world and the next. For example, I see a man whose eyes are closed, is only able to lie in bed, is unable to eat or drink and has no observable responses to his environment. He doesn't appear to be participating in any way in this realm and yet he is not moving on into death.

I think: Why isn't he dying? What is keeping him here? What could he still need? As I did with Mrs. Jenkins (page 213), I can tend to project my own thoughts and angst onto him, assuming that he is suffering and experiencing unfinished business that needs to come to resolution. At times, this may be the case. However, I want to emphasize that for us to lock into our rational thinking with continual assessment and worry is probably the least helpful thing for the person with dementia. His process, whatever it may be, will unfold with or without our over-analyzing it. I am convinced of this. In each case, I may not have fully understood how the process played out, but countless times I have witnessed the transformation. The most helpful stance for me and the person with dementia is to return to the basics of being in the rhythm of connection.

JUANITA

Juanita climbed very high on the corporate ladder. She was efficient, strong and committed to helping other women rise in nontraditional business positions. When she found out that she had a brain tumor at the age of 62, she negotiated a consultant position so she could put most of her energies into fighting the tumor. After eighteen months, three surgeries, multiple rounds of radiation and chemotherapy, Juanita said, "I have lost this battle. It is time." She said she was ready to die.

She and I spent several weeks putting all of her affairs in order. Some days she was clear-thinking, other days she had difficulty expressing thoughts and finding words, but she succeeded in not only tying up all her loose ends, but also tying bows on Christmas packages she intended for family and friends after she was gone.

Juanita peacefully and quietly waited for November 17th, only eight more days—the day her mother died five years before, the day Juanita knew she would also die. As you might imagine, we talked a lot about time lines, expectations and disappointments, but she firmly referenced her female intuition as her source of understanding.

November 17th was one great day. Juanita's three adult children gathered around her bed and friends and business acquaintances filed in and out of her room to say their good-byes. All was orchestrated according to her plan. The day came and went as usual, and so did the following week. Juanita was confused at first, then irritated with God for not respecting her plan; this rapidly escalated into a tortured state of rage at God for not wanting her in heaven, after all. "Who is He to keep me out!?" she shouted. She repeatedly reminded all of us that she had a very impressive resume, enumerating her qualifications so we would agree that she be allowed her spot in heaven. Her rage turned toward everyone around her. She was infuriated that she had not died and was not dying. "I'm not going to stand for this treatment," she shouted day and night. She refused any spiritual counselors, her priest or anyone who tried to speak rationally with her.

Juanita did allow me to stay with her if I quietly sat and listened to her vent. And so I did, as I continued to work personally on holding a nonjudgmental, compassionate and open heart to the pain in her struggle. My presence at least helped to release some of that pressure for the rest of the day, but it resurfaced the next. Each day Juanita shifted into longer periods of a semi-restful sleep—rarely did her fidgeting or frown disappear. Whenever she awakened, her old clear-thinking, raging self returned.

The only change occurred on December 2nd, when Juanita moved the target of her rage from God to her mother: "Where the hell is she when I need her?!" I asked if she had seen her mother recently and her eyes threw fire as she screamed, "I'M NOT CRAZY! SHE'S DEAD! OF COURSE I HAVEN'T SEEN HER!" I said I knew she wasn't crazy and that a lot of people toward the end of life see people who had died. Those people aren't crazy either!

With that statement, Juanita relaxed and her demeanor became calm and focused. For the first time since November 17th she was open, curious and fully present with me. She asked for examples of what some others had experienced, and I gave her many. She told me that she had a vision of her mother the night before and she thought she was totally losing it. Her mother talked with her and said that, "It will be a bit longer, my dear one." She also told Juanita, "Use this time to be kind with others. Use it well and I will be here with open arms when you come." From this moment forward, she held her mother's words with her, literally written on an index card so she would not forget. Juanita remained pleasant, peaceful and loving until her final breath on December 20th.

FRITZIE

Fritzie was a gentle, loving man who had married Beth after her first husband's death. He became an extraordinary father to Beth's ten children. The love they all showed him throughout his 11-year decline was a beautiful testimony to him. When his needs required a skilled care facility, they worked out a schedule to remain actively present for him, even though many lived very far away. Parishioners from his church came by daily to read from his prayer book or bible and to shake his hand.

His hands were large and strong. His eyes had quiet depth that drew people in and gave them permission to relax, settle in and be with him for a while. He rarely spoke, and when he did, it was usually a simple "yes" or "no" to a question. A "no" stated a clear preference, but he said "yes" to just about everything else. According to his family, that is how he lived his life—with a big "YES."

In the course of a month, Fritzie had another series of small strokes that brought him to the next level of decline and he was unable to take in any food or water. About 10 years before he had drawn up a living will which his family now honored—they did not have a feeding tube placed. The physician met with Beth to tell her that Fritzie probably only had a few more days of life. She immediately called all the family to come to say their final good-byes. Unfortunately, two sons in the armed forces overseas would probably not return in time. Everybody else flew in from all over the country to be present in whatever ways they could—for their father, for their mother and for each other.

During the next eight days, Fritzie lost even more weight, did not speak and when he did open his eyes he stared off into the distance. All the professional staff wondered how his endurance was possible because he had so few physical reserves even before his recent strokes. He had seen everyone in his life during those eight days—even the two sons from overseas were able to get home. Everyone made beautiful closure with him, individually and collectively. How could he still be here...or why? Then, we put the questioning aside and brought ourselves back to being fully present with him.

On the ninth day, finally the entire family was in the facility at the same time. Twenty-six people crammed into Fritzie's room! One daughter said her dad, "came back to life when we surrounded him with all this love." He was certainly weak, but he opened his eyes and focused on each person in that room and gave a gentle smile and nod of his head.

Then, he did something that stunned us all. He took his wife's hand into his left hand, reached out into what we perceived as empty space to take something with his right hand and placed it into his wife's hand, enclosing them between his large hands. He then performed this ritual with each of his 10 children. Everyone was in tears with the beauty of this gesture. It was as if Fritzie matched up each person with a guardian angel or introduced each to a presence from his or her lineage. When Fritzie completed each gesture, he relaxed back into his pillow. Everyone in the room joined hands in prayers of thanks for the gifts received and for the beauty this man brought to the world. During the prayer, Fritzie took his last breath, his apparent desire for making these unexplainable connections having been fulfilled.

CATHY

It was hard to understand what Cathy was saying most of the time. We had to listen very carefully for the themes that emerged briefly between her nonsensical wordings. She was living with her husband who was her caregiver in their home of 43 years. It had not been an easy six years since Cathy's diagnosis of Alzheimer's disease, but her husband remained committed to keeping her at home. He accepted occasional help from their son and two daughters who, although they were willing, were inundated with their own busy schedules. Even so, about once every two weeks he was able to take a day to himself, to help preserve some of his sanity, he said.

Our hospice services got a call from Cathy's husband two weeks after a big family gathering. During a particularly clear-minded day for Cathy, she had asked for the get-together. On the day of the event, Cathy said her final good-byes to them all. According to her husband it was a great day full of light-hearted stories, laughter, very loving memories and tears. "The following day," he said, "Cathy stopped eating and began to just fade away but not with a whole lot of peace." He told us that Cathy was increasingly very upset, but the family was having trouble understanding what to do to help her.

When I met with Cathy she was still upset, frequently bringing herself to tears while trying to tell me what was going on, what was worrying her. She was quite animated—waving her arms and making faces to supplement all the missing words. The themes I picked up on were very clear—it was about her going "there" or staying in "this" place and whichever she did, "they" would be upset, which she indicated by frowning and looking very sad. No matter what, she was bound to upset someone she cared about. She held my hands and kept asking me, "What?" and "How?"

What suddenly popped into my head was Beth, whom I had accompanied during her struggles a few years earlier. I remembered sitting at Beth's bedside during the last few days of her life and looking up above her fireplace at a pencil sketch of ducks flying in formation. I commented on the beauty of the picture but Beth shook her head and said, "Migration is such a dirty business." Beth was in that struggle between worlds—to stay here is to disappoint all the people "over there" who are welcoming her with "open arms." To go with "them" will "hurt everyone here."

As Beth's story popped into my head, I found myself saying to Cathy, "Yeah...migration is such a dirty business." Cathy laughed instantly and repeated several times, "Migration is such a dirty business." She latched onto that phrase and said it to everyone who came to see her, each time laughing and nodding her head in agreement. For reasons I will never understand, this hit the spot and certainly helped to transform her angst in that moment. Even when she would slip back into upset, her husband and family could bring her back to that transformative place by helping her to remember this simple phrase. It became the family's mantra. Cathy began to eat again and to fully take in the support and love that was coming to her from so many directions. She blossomed and lived for two more years, laughing, smiling and graciously entertaining all who came to visit her.

At times, we see the person with dementia having moments of connection with something or someone in that expanded field of energy or the other side. There seems to be a definite and precise process even if the person has profound dementia and whether or not we ever fully perceive or understand how it occurs. It could be the person's first exposure and he might need some extra time to become familiar or comfortable with these encounters with the expanded field. He might want to help make connections between loved ones on this side of life with those he perceives on the other side of this life. He may need to hear from someone he trusts that everything is okay and that he is exactly where he should be in that moment, doing exactly what he needs to do. Perhaps he has been such a strong survivor throughout life that his body doesn't quite know the meaning of the word "enough." I could go on for pages with guesses as to what the process is that leads one to finally letting go. In the end, they would still only be guesses.

To maintain peaceful curiosity and gentle exploration can be fine, but never at the cost of losing the loving connection in those moments with the person who has dementia as he progresses through whatever is his process. As he gets closer and closer to his final moments, his connections will frequently shift, sometimes gradually or sometimes rather abruptly, away from those of us in this life and toward representations of the next life. Our stance is to accept without judgment his new connections and awarenesses, and remain available to him in loving presence, wherever he is in that moment. By doing this, we will encourage his openness, and support him through the final moments of his transition into death.

FINAL MOMENTS OF TRANSITION

I have been blessed with hundreds of opportunities to be available during those last moments as a person makes her transition from life to death. I am constantly in awe of the wisdom in the timing of some persons' deaths. A person could have been nonresponsive, unable to have a rational thought in years, or seem incapable of taking in any information from the world around him—yet she slid into death at what seemed to me the most synchronistic moment:

- when her favorite hymn or song was playing on a CD;
- when a priest was administering the Sacrament of the Sick, a rabbi was providing a blessing, Buddhists were chanting, a shaman was drumming;
- when her closest friend or relative came in to hold her hand and just finished telling her how much she was loved;
- when a counselor had just walked into the room and would be available to support the grieving process of a son or daughter the dying person felt was the most fragile;
- when that last family member just walked out the door after a beautiful and joyous day spent celebrating the person's life.

What are the odds? These things happen with amazing regularity. The timing sometimes is just too exact to be a coincidence. There must be a greater wisdom working here, or so it seems.

The Timing of Death

Whatever the timing of death, I have learned that it is most certainly not within my control. My first confrontation with this reality happened way back when I was a teenager and believed that no one should ever die alone. A person very dear to me, Kitty, had been pronounced brain dead from a head trauma and she lay dying in the hospital. I stayed with her for 32 straight hours, mostly holding her hand. A couple of times I bent forward and caught a little nap by her side, but the moment came in the middle of the night when I just HAD to have a cup of coffee. I told Kitty, in case she could understand, that I was going down the hall for some coffee. I was gone for no more than three minutes...honestly...and darned if she didn't die while I was out. I vacillated between guilt for not being there for her and irritation, thinking "Not for nothing...you couldn't have waited a minute 'til I got back?"

I finally decided that this really is about her, after all. Perhaps she needed to die without me there; perhaps it was harder to let go with such a dear friend present. Perhaps she was protecting me or herself from the pain of the separation of that moment—or none of the above. Who knows? I certainly did learn that none of it was within my control and that it really wasn't about me.

I've also learned that the timing of death is beyond my assumptions, a lesson I received from being with two persons with dementia who died, one right after the other.

MR. MILLER

His physician told me that Mr. Miller showed all the signs of actively dying—his legs were mottled from toe to knee, which indicated that his heart was shutting down. His breathing was irregular and he was no longer responding even to uncomfortable stimuli. The physician thought Mr. Miller had only a few more hours of life left, and asked me to contact his daughter. The daughter was trapped in a hurricane in

Florida and could not get a plane for two days. I returned to the room and called the daughter from Mr. Miller's telephone so she could talk to her father and say what she needed to say—even though he was not responsive. Our hope was that he would still be able to take in information on some level, of course. I remained as available to him as possible for that day, the next day, and for part of the day after that when his daughter walked into the room. Beyond all medical odds, Mr. Miller had been able to last long enough for his daughter to be present with him. He died fifteen minutes after she got there.

RUTH

That same afternoon, in another room down the hall, Ruth was dying and I was, once again, asked to call the daughter to come in. Ruth was not showing any active signs of dying but she was minimally responsive and stopped taking in any food. The best 'guestimate' by her physician was that she had somewhere between several days to maybe a week of life left—certainly enough time for the daughter to fly in from California. I called the daughter and made the arrangements—she would be coming in to see her mother the next morning. I went to Ruth's room and told her of her daughter's arrival time and I sat with her. Because of the experience with Mr. Miller, I just assumed that Ruth would hang in there until her daughter came, but within ten minutes, Ruth very peacefully slipped away.

Probably because Ruth's and Mr. Miller's deaths were so closely timed, the situations so similar, and yet the resolve so opposite, I very clearly got it that I cannot assume or predict anyone's timing of death. When I can relax, give my inquiring and assuming mind a coffee break and remain present with openness and love, I allow her the space and give her the support to do what she needs to do— how ever it plays out.

The timing of a person's death often makes total sense in hindsight, interestingly enough. In looking back, I was glad that Kitty didn't die while I was in the room—I was more frightened of that moment of death in those days than I was willing to admit. Mr. Miller's daughter knew he would hang on for her to get there. He had been dependent on her for emotional support for the past forty years and always said he would need her help when the time comes. And Ruth's daughter was saddened by her mother's death but also lovingly reminisced that, "Well, wasn't that ever my Mom...always was an independent cuss!"

We often work at making sense of the unique timing and process of the person's death in hindsight because finding meaning is self-comforting in our grief. Perhaps the dying person with dementia has the same instinctual wisdom about when to leave this world as she somehow had as to when to enter it. Or, maybe the wisdom in the timing comes from the loving connections—both in corporeal form and in the extended field— that surround the person making that final transition. A greater wisdom may allow everything to unfold in the way that is most healing for both the person who is dying and those around her, even though such wisdom and healing might not be immediately apparent to any of us. It could be a combination of all these possibilities—it really is a both-and, not an either-or universe. We each will come to our own, very individual understandings with each series of events that lead to death.

Intuition

The more time I spend with persons who have dementia in each one's final moments, the more aware I become of my own intuition. In this sense, I use the word intuition to mean "inner knowing"—knowledge in the heart as opposed to the mind; knowledge that is evidenced when we focus on what we "hear" when listening with the heart. There is nothing mystical about sensing what is appropriate with a person, with or without dementia, even if he is not responsive or interactive. Intuition is a matter of merely noting what claims your attention. It may not make rational sense, but it grabs your heart or gut.

Many of us who work in hospice have had countless experiences of one of our clients suddenly popping into our thoughts as we are going through our scheduled day. At times, I have such a strong sense of the person that I change my schedule in order to visit him that very day, or in the next moment, only to find that he has taken a sudden turn and is now actively dying. At other times, I might put off seeing him, only to find out that he died at the time he came into my thoughts. That news can make me sad that I didn't respond to my intuition; but then I realize that I definitely was with him at his time of death—I was holding him with loving thoughts in my heart during his transition.

Family members often tell stories of just happening to change their plans and drop by unexpectedly, to find their loved one's condition suddenly changed and death imminent.

We often dismiss this inner knowing as mere coincidence, until we acknowledge the frequency and uncanny timing of events. This leads us to validate and use them in caregiving. Sometimes, the intuitive hit is so wildly beyond the possibility of coincidence that denial is pointless.

NORA

Nora was a woman I visited a few times over a period of about six weeks. She had profound dementia due to a series of small strokes that occurred over a twelve-year period. She was totally dependent on caregivers, but was still capable of establishing eye contact, holding hands and smiling every now and then. She became more alert while connecting with three specific people—her spiritual counselor, our expressive puppetry professional and me—but her capacity to interact remained severely limited.

One morning, Nora was very much on my mind, but I tried not to be distracted as I tried to continue my tasks of the day. Within an hour, the hospice nurse paged me to say that Nora had taken a turn the night before, that it was probably another stroke. She was taking in no nutrition and totally unresponsive. No one had been able to contact the only surviving daughter at that point. The hospice nurse asked me to go to the facility to help staff with this sudden change in condition—they had helped Nora for over 10 years and those who were very connected to her were having a difficult time.

I met with the staff in Nora's room, which allowed them to talk about their memories and their connections with this woman over the years. Their greatest wish, as they expressed it, was for me to spend some time with Nora, to give her extra TLC and to help in whatever ways she needed. So, I sat with Nora, holding her hand and quietly being with her. She lay very still on her bed; her only movement came in irregular breaths with twenty second periods of apnea (not breathing) every minute. Her eyes remained closed and she did not respond when I hugged or touched her hand.

All of a sudden, an up-tempo tune, reminiscent of Gaelic music of some kind, popped into my head. It struck me as very odd because it was such a perky, snappy little ditty. I just couldn't get it out of my head, so I decided to hum it out loud. I hoped no one else could hear me because even I judged this as a bit over the edge—bizarre for a death-bed scene.

I had been humming the tune for about five minutes when suddenly Nora opened her eyes and leaned forward into a half-sitting position. She stared off, focused keenly on what appeared to be a vision and said quite softly and respectfully, "Anna." I kept singing. Then she smiled, laid back into her bed, closed her eyes and took a long, deep sigh—her last breath.

Later on, Nora's daughter told me that her mother had another daughter, who had died 54 years earlier. Her name was Anna. As her daughter reminisced about her mother, I heard that Nora was raised in an Irish community in Canada and was passionate about her culture and Gaelic music. After that conversation, I could no longer easily dismiss this or any intuition as coincidence. What seemed to be looking me in the face was that this inner knowing, or intuitive hit, as I like to call it, was from some wisdom beyond my rational abilities to explain or understand.

When I sit with the person with dementia who is near death, those unexplainable thoughts or hunches most often claim my attention through the heart with a feeling. This happens especially when outside distractions and interruptions are few, and opportunities for shared silence and for simply being with are many. At times, I sense a presence in the room with us, only to see the person with dementia look with awe at something that remains invisible to me. At other times, a phrase, expression or a poem will pop into my head while I am with a person who has dementia. More often than not, his loved ones later tell me that my sudden thought described his essence, the way he lived his life.

Sometimes, while sitting with a dying person, in one moment I am filled with emotional warmth and overwhelming gratitude and in the next, the person tries to tell me of his vision of heaven as he is seeing it. At other times, I feel that a presence is standing behind me touching my shoulders and passing tingling, healing energies through me toward the person I am embracing, only to have that person take his last, deep and peaceful breath in that moment. And almost always, I feel the most profound sense of love that envelopes the person as he makes that final transition from this more limited life into the expanded field.

Hundreds of people have shared with me their own experiences over the last 20 years—some experiences being quite similar to mine, some beautifully unique. We all have intuitions and the ability to be present and open to them. As human beings, we are wired with this other way of knowing and accessing the quiet wisdom that is present within and around us. The more I have paid attention to all those little hunches and synchronicities that occur during my day, the less shy I have become about following through or taking action. And the time between intuition and action has become both shorter and less fraught with doubt or self-judgment.

Intuition is innate and everyone's ability to be intuitive will be strengthened as we pay attention and rehearse opening to it. Reacquainting yourself with the exercise from Chapter 5 entitled "Keep Track of the Little 'Hits'" in *Expand Your Awareness* can be helpful in stretching your intuitive awarenesses. I encourage you to open to the possibilities, to pay attention with all of your senses and to observe the great resources that occur within each moment.

SUMMARY

The person with dementia experiences death in millions of tiny losses during what is often a long and slow deterioration. We have an extraordinary opportunity to connect as his time on this earth plays out and the final moment of death occurs. To do so requires us to keep looking within. Do I have any internal barriers, opinions, judgments or expectations that interfere with my abilities to remain fully present, in inner silence and love in each moment? Can I open to the potential of the person with dementia to participate in decision-making and in end-of-life processing? Can I find ways that can help him come to closure with this life? Am I able to remain open to the possibility that the person with dementia can participate in the processing that supports his transition at the end of life?

Certainly, not every scenario is tranquil as the person with dementia makes the final transition into death. However, in the vast majority of my experiences at a person's final moments, I have seen a tangible shift manifest—perhaps as a very deep level of relaxation, an expression of relief or of great comfort or a look of peace. Sometimes before and/or after the moment of death, the person is radiant—with an energy that is spiritual, not physical. I often am stunned by the realization that the dying person—who we so recently perceived as losing everything—is in the throes of a huge caring, loving even joyful event. Could these persons with dementia be experiencing what saints and sages have described through the ages?

These observations led me to generalize my understanding that the psychological, emotional and spiritual transformation of the person with dementia can not only still occur but be facilitated and encouraged by our supportive ability to remain an inwardly silent, open and loving presence. I may never really understand how this occurs—and today, I can let go of that need to understand. I 'just' get to witness these miraculous transformations happen—to everyday persons like you and me.

Love is the bridge—our loving presence is our bond with the love that the person with dementia perceives and interacts with in the expanded field of energy. Love is his final connection with this life and at the door that opens into the next. Love has the capacity to reach beyond all those years of physical deterioration and exhaustion of spirit, to open the person with dementia to this transformation.

WORKING IT OUT

Begin your own life review and increase your comfort in being with persons at the end of life.

Your Five Wishes

I strongly suggest you order several copies of the *Five Wishes* booklet from Aging with Dignity by calling the toll free 1-888-5-WISHES number (594-7437), or by visiting *www.agingwithdignity.org*. Very easy to use and understand, *Five Wishes* is the first living will with a heart. It goes beyond medical decision-making to encourage thinking about your personal, emotional and spiritual needs. What is most important is that it supports dialogue between you and your family, friends and doctors. Much of the guesswork and uncertainties are removed, leaving you and your loved one more available to be fully present in the time of need.

When your family members talk about their advance directives and fill out their individual *Five Wishes* forms together, it takes the spotlight pressure off the ill person. Discussions and choices about end-of-life care are important for everyone to make, not simply the currently ill or declining person. This family-inclusive way of talking it over helps everybody feel less defensive and more willing to participate. For some families, it also can be helpful to elicit the aid of a willing close friend, a social worker, physician or other helping professional to open the door to the discussions.

Do Your Own Spiritual Inventory

In her excellent presentation on understanding and effectively managing end-of-life issues, Enid Schwartz provides questions that help guide a person through his own spiritual inventory. This is a valuable exercise for any one of us at any point in life. Once again, get comfortable and relaxed. Try to honor each question with an adequate amount of time, with your full attention and with honest reflection.

- How have you used your gift of human life?
- What do you need to 'clear up' or 'let go of' to be more peaceful?

- What gives your life meaning?
- For what are you grateful?
- What have you learned of love and how well have you learned to love?
- What have you learned of tenderness, vulnerability, intimacy and communion?
- What have you learned about courage, strength, power and faith?
- How are you handling your suffering?
- What helps you open your heart and empty your mind so that you can experience the presence of Spirit?
- What will give you strength as you die?
- If you remembered that your breaths were numbered, what would be your relationship with your breath right now?
- If I were to ask you who you are, what would be your response?

[Reprinted with permission from materials presented in a workshop sponsored by PESI Healthcare, LLC. © 2001 by Enid Schwartz.]

Write Your Own Obituary

This might strike you as morbid, but it is an excellent exercise for looking at your life and acknowledging your accomplishments. What do you want people to remember about you? What are you most proud of? What do you really love about yourself? How has the world become a better place because you participated in it? Try to stretch beyond "Just the facts, Ma'am" into providing a true reflection on who you have been and what will live beyond your physical body. Spend a focused amount of time on this exercise to help clarify and validate your life's purpose.

Bring More Awareness to the Dying Process

In *The Book of Secrets*, Deepak Chopra talks about how prayer, rituals, meditation and assistance from the living can help shift the dying person's perception from this experience is happening to me to I am creating this experience. When we bring more awareness to the dying process, we rid ourselves of excessive fear and anxiety.

One way of increasing your awareness of the person's dying process is to spend some serious time with your full attention in reflection about the person's life. Since the person who has dementia is quite possibly unable to participate in a direct discussion, imagine having a conversation with him. Yes, imagine sitting in some overstuffed chairs in a quiet room with a fireplace and talking over a cup of coffee, or walking with him in the woods as you did when you were a child. In whatever calming place you choose to place the two of you, allow to come to surface some honest reflections on how this man lived his life.

- Talk with him about his good memories, accomplishments and successes in life. Ask, what has been most meaningful and filled him with gratitude. Share with him what it has been about his life that has most touched your heart.

- Ask what he has learned of love, courage, vulnerability, strength, intimacy, power, communion and faith. Share with him what he has taught you about these things.
- Ask him to talk about what has given him strength and helped open his heart and empty his mind so he could experience the presence of Spirit or a power greater than himself. Share with him how he has expanded your awarenesses. Maybe he has provided you with strength and opened your heart. Perhaps acknowledging his presence in your life will help you to know that he will always be with you, that you will never be alone.

Imagining this talk will require you to reach down into yourself. Powerful feelings might surface, and as you accept and deal with them you will become more available to the person with dementia who is dying. Many of your awarenesses certainly can be audibly reflected to him when you next see him. As I experienced with Fannie Wheeler, expressing your reflections may be exactly what he needs to fully accept his life and let go with an open spirit.

Imagining this talk is also effective if the person has already died, particularly if death occurred before you had a chance to say whatever you needed to say.

To totally stretch yourself, you can also imagine having this dialogue with yourself at the end of life.

8 – Beyond Remembering

In the fall of 2002, I joined a small group of women for a retreat at a beautiful home in New Hampshire. Each of us had been actively involved in relief efforts after the 9/11 attacks in New York City and we were gathering to network, nurture, support and hopefully inspire each other. I was looking forward to an enriching time—long walks in the White Mountains at the peak of fall foliage, meeting new people from diverse and fascinating backgrounds and creating culinary delights; I had been designated connoisseur of chocolate.

Unfortunately, the pressing need for individual healing dominated the weekend and the time I had hoped for igniting and uplifting my spirit just did not happen. By departure time Sunday, I was more drained than when I had arrived. I had listened to one too many stories about ongoing physically and emotionally abusive relationships, about who was having affairs with whom, and about multiple levels of betrayal and lack of integrity in personal and professional lives.

I focused intensely on reaching for connections with each person, on withholding my opinions and judgments in order to see from the story teller's perspective and on keeping a loving inner silence as I opened to thankfulness for our time together. There were a few moments of connection for me, but for the most part, I worked very hard all weekend when I REALLY needed a break from neediness.

On the drive home, I spiraled into judgment and anger. How could Ann, Mary Ellen and Ginger allow the abuse from their husbands to go on and on? Why were these intelligent women staying in crazy relationships? How could Stella and Barbara be capable of such compassionate action, especially throughout the previous year, yet live with incongruity, infidelity and blatant disdain and disregard for themselves and, at times, for others? Then, of course, my judgments turned on me! Why couldn't Ms. Compassionate Listener take a weekend off? How insecure or stupid was I to not clearly own and state *my* needs for nurturing and healing? What role did *I* play in feeling dumped on?

To put it mildly, my buttons were stuck in the pushed position! By the time I got home, my relentless mental and emotional spiral had sucked many of my own significant life relationships into the black current of my thinking. There were those family members and many close friends who vented anger and spewed negative judgments instead of dealing with diversity or change, sometimes foisting hurtful accusations on me. I enumerated all the betrayals and abuse. I remembered how I too, chose to hang on way beyond the unhealthy point. I went on and on, reclaiming all the dark emotions from my 53 years and successfully buried myself under a pile of self-directed judgment and anger.

Then, I began to hate myself for being so angry and judgmental. I knew better! I knew that I was partly responsible for the rampant anger in the world when I lingered in this state but I didn't seem to have the ability to shift out of it. I vacillated between understanding everyone else and justifying my anger and judgment against them and myself. I felt as though my mind was short circuiting, creating random glitches of near-insight that illuminated nothing even as I was desperate for the clarity to make sense of something—anything to get me relief from my disgusting feelings. Practicing focused breathing and meditating, and giving myself a Reiki treatment, only provided temporary release from my racing mind and heart. Taking a shower didn't wash anything away. So I decided to see if I could walk it off.

As I walked, I tried to practice the six basic **IF LOST** principles that you have read about in this book and persons with dementia had helped me live—heaven knew I certainly *felt* lost! Perhaps I could let them help me as they so often had, to resolve my current state.

Nope. I was too far gone. I couldn't even pretend to want to connect with those whom I was sure did not even care about living in a loving way. My attempts at a loving inner silence were completely bombarded by my justification for rage and intolerance of the way human beings treat one another. Thankfulness was a principle I couldn't even spell in that moment! I was truly tortured. I needed some form of insight that would help me move forward with loving acceptance of myself and the other people trapped inside the chaotic disease of my anger.

My mind flashed to Sara, the woman whose dementia was so profound yet whose heart was always filled with joy and gratitude (Chapter 6, page 181). I saw myself in that moment as sharing something in common with Sara. We each had very chaotic conditions—hers being dementia, mine being anger—and each of us was incapable of being able to work anything out rationally. But Sara was beyond remembering all the struggles of her life and lived in the present moment, filled with grace.

I closed my eyes as I continued to walk in full stride and I focused on reaching out beyond myself and my short circuited half-truths. I wanted so much to bring myself into a space like Sara's—beyond remembering. In my desperation, I put away my need to figure it all out on my own and instead placed all of my attention on surrendering to what was and opening my heart to the unknown. I reached beyond myself with a wholehearted plea for some form of connection to something—anything outside myself that would help bring me just a little sense of that joy and gratitude Sara so beautifully embodied.

Dozens of strides later, I suddenly came to a full stop and opened my eyes. There in front of me, about six feet away, was a mother skunk leading her four little baby skunks across the road. I knew in an instant that I received the answer to my plea. Those five little creatures in front of me were there to let me know that these people whom I judged so fiercely—including myself—were simply *skunks*!

Well, this thoroughly appealed to my sense of humor; I was tickled beyond belief. I KNEW there was a great humor out there in the expanded field of energy! Along with my delight came a release and permission to treat myself less seriously and more gently.

Of course, that wasn't the only message in the synchronistic encounter with the skunks. I also understood in that moment that skunks have a unique and particularly nasty defense system; I was certainly glad I hadn't bumped into them literally. But when skunks are not threatened and in defense mode, they are beautiful, cuddly and easy to admire and love.

The message came across loud and clear: People are like skunks. When we perceive danger, we activate our defenses, which can manifest at times in a variety of repugnant ways. I can choose to interact with others so as to try to minimize their need for defenses; I can choose to simply give them a wide berth. Whatever the case, their defenses are merely that and they do not alter the person's essential beauty.

Everything fell into place. Seeing the skunks gave me the insight to see all human beings in all the cute "fluffiness" and innocence with which we were born. It allowed me to return to love and thankfulness for all the people who have been in my life, regardless of how they manifested. It allowed me to open again to self-love and thankfulness for the gift of something that was always there but somehow spontaneously emerged in my awareness.

I was stunned by the fact that nothing changed except how I looked at the situations and relationships in my life—as though I simply put on a different pair of glasses and for the first time could magically see the essential beauty inside everything.

Suddenly, I remembered a phrase I had read in Stuart Kaufman's *At Home in the Universe*: order emerges at the edge of chaos. I was experiencing a sense of order on this side of my own chaos. My mind quickly accumulated countless examples of how order emerged for me while connecting with persons who have dementia over the years. When I do not attend to the chaos of the disease's impact and instead, bring a clear focus to connecting with the person who has dementia, there is a supporting and encouraging of the order and the strengths that exist within her. As I pay closer attention, I see more and more manifestations of this order. I have also come to understand that there is a greater order in the expanded field of energy—what some call the realm of spirit—that I may never see manifested. Still, I know it exists. This is not just a matter of blind faith. As I practice *being with* and as I connect to persons with dementia, my heart understands.

I am not the same person as when I began my journey. I have changed. It has been through my relationships with persons who have dementia that I have been given the gifts of grasping and living the wisdom inherent in the six basic **IF LOST** spiritual and religious principles discussed in this book. By focusing my attention on exploring connections, I not only discovered my personal barriers and resistances but unearthed unexpected hidden strengths that I had been afraid to claim. I gradually became open and willing to remain vulnerable, genuine and nondefensive as I looked at the world through new eyes. I was led into unknown territories that challenged and stretched both my adaptability and integrity while expanding my taste for magic, mystery, wonder and delight in all connections. I was given countless opportunities to experience compassion and love—for myself and others—while opening to and trusting ongoing interactions with the expanded field of energy.

I began my work knowing that my opportunity was to be present with persons who have dementia in such a way as to encourage each person to continue to participate in life. I found in the process that I also was participating in life more than ever before. This has been the beauty of connection for me—each of us was able to see the other and feel seen by the other; each of us moved beyond isolation; each of us was empowered to move forward, to grow. We have guided, encouraged, inspired and accompanied each other in connection—with ourselves, each other, the world around us and the expanded field of energy. Each of us transformed in the single moment of connection; each of us changed in the most miniscule and grand ways forever.

APPENDIX

CHAPTER REFERENCES

Chapter 1 - Introduction

Kaplan, Alexandra. "The 'Self-in-Relation;' Implications for Depression in Women," in *Women's Growth in Connection,* Jordan, et al. (New York: Guilford Press, 1991)

Lionel, Frédéric. Conference entitled *Messages of the Western Mystic Tradition in Their Present Day Applications* (Bore Place Commonwork Center, England: 1990)

Mace, Nancy L. and Peter V. Rabins. *The 36-Hour Day* (New York: Warner Books, 1999)

Miller, Jean Baker. *Toward a New Psychology of Women* (2nd ed.) (Boston: Beacon Press, 1986)

Miller, Jean Baker. Work in Progress #33: "Connections, Disconnections and Violations" (Wellesley, MA: The Stone Center, 1988)

Miller, Jean Baker and Irene Pierce Stiver. *The Healing Connection: How Women Form Relationships in Therapy and Life* (Boston: Beacon Press, 1997)

Chapter 2 - Intend a Connection

Chopra, Deepak. *The Seven Spiritual Laws of Success* (CA: Amber-Allen/New World Library, 1994)

Dyer, Wayne. *The Power of Intention* (Hay House, 2004)

Myss, Caroline. *Caroline Myss' Essential Guide for Healers* (CO: Sounds True, 2004) 4 CDs

Toms, Michael and Justin Willis Toms. *True Work: Doing What You Love and Loving What You Do* (New York: Bell Tower, 1998)

Chapter 3 – Free Yourself
of Opinions and Judgments

Lionel, Frédéric. Conference entitled *Messages of the Western Mystic Tradition in Their Present Day Applications* (Bore Place Commonwork Center, England: 1990)

Prather, Hugh. *The Little Book of Letting Go: A Revolutionary 30-Day Program to Cleanse your Mind, Lift your Spirit and Replenish your Soul* (Boston: Conari Press, 2000)

Walsh, Robert. Essential Spirituality: *Exercises from the World's Religions to Cultivate Kindness, Love, Joy, Peace, Vision, Wisdom, and Generosity* (New York: John Wiley & Sons, Inc., 1999)

Writer's Workshop Residents. "The World is not Black and White." *JHA* 𝍇 (New Haven, CT: JHA, Spring, 1989)

Chapter 4 – Love and Open
to Being Loved

Childre, Doc and Howard Martin. *The HeartMath Solution* (San Francisco: HarperCollins Publishers, 1999)

Childre, Doc and Deborah Rozman. *Transforming Stress: The HeartMath Solution for Relieving Worry, Fatigue, and Tension* (CA: New Harbinger Publications, Inc., 2005)

Coste, Joanne Koenig. *Learning to Speak Alzheimer's: A Groundbreaking Approach For Everyone Dealing with the Disease* (Boston: Houghton Mifflin Company, 2003)

Denney, Ann. "Quiet Music: An Intervention for Mealtime Agitation" in *Journal of Gerontological Nursing.* Vol. 23(7): July, 1997.

Germain, Carel B. *Social Work Practice in Health Care: An Ecological Perspective* (New York: The Free Press, 1984)

Germain, Carel B. and Alex Gitterman. *The Life Model of Social Work Practice* (New York: Columbia University Press, 1980)

Hatfield, Agnes and H. Lefley. *Families of the Mentally Ill: Coping and Adaptation* (New York: Guilford, 1987)

Lionel, Frédéric. Conference entitled *Messages of the Western Mystic Tradition in Their Present Day Applications* (Bore Place Commonwork Center, England: 1990)

Miller, Jean Baker and Irene Pierce Stiver. *The Healing Connection: How Women Form Relationships in Therapy and in Life* (Boston, Beacon Press, 1997)

Murphy, Lois B. and Alice Moriarty. *Vulnerability, coping, and growth: From infancy to adolescence* (CT, Yale University Press, 1978)

Chapter 5 – Silence and the Art of Being With the Person who has Dementia

Cameron, Julia. *The Artist's Way: A Spiritual Path to Higher Creativity* (New York: J. P. Tarcher, 2002)

Harper, Tim. *The Uncommon Touch: An Investigation of Spiritual Healing* (Ontario: McClelland & Steward Inc., 1994)

Jordan, Judith. Work in Progress #16: "Empathy and Self Boundaries" (Wellesley, MA: Stone Center, 1984)

Jordan Judith. Work in Progress #102: "Valuing Vulnerability: New Definitions of Courage" (Wellesley, MA: Stone Center, 2003)

Lionel, Frédéric. Conference entitled *Messages of the Western Mystic Tradition in Their Present Day Applications* (Bore Place Commonwork Center, England: 1990)

Miller, J. B. Work in Progress #22: "What Do We Mean by Relationships?" (Wellesley, MA: Stone Center, 1986)

Miller, J. B. and I. P. Stiver. *The Healing Connection: How Women Form Relationships in Therapy and Life* (Boston: Beacon Press, 1997)

Schneider, Marge. *A Hand in Healing: The Power of Expressive Puppetry* (Anticipated Publication 2007)

Surrey, Janet. Work in Progress #13: "Self-in-Relation: A Theory of Women's Development" (Wellesley, MA: Stone Center, 1985)

Warner, M. L. *The Complete Guide to Alzheimer's-Proofing Your Home* (Rev. ed.) (Indiana: Purdue University Press, 2000)

Chapter 6 - Thankfulness

Vernon, Rama J. "Gratitude: An Unspoken, Silent Prayer," in *Gratitude: A Way of Life,* Louise L. Hay and Friends (CA: Hay House, Inc., 1996)

Walsh, Roger. *Essential Spirituality: The 7 Central Practices to Awaken Heart and Mind* (NY: John Wiley & Sons, Inc., 1999)

Writer's Workshop Residents. "Dealing with Stress." *JHA* 𝕿𝕿 (New Haven: JHA, Fall, 1990)

Chapter 7 – Connections at the End of Life

Aging with Dignity. *Five Wishes* (1-888-594-7437 or www.agingwithdignity.org)

Butler, Robert N. "Successful Aging and the Role of the Life Review." *Journal of American Geriatric Society* 22 (1974): 529-35.

Chopra, Deepak. *The Book of Secrets: Unlocking the Hidden Dimensions of Your Life* (NY: Three Rivers Press, 2004)

Levine, Stephen. *Healing into Life and Death* (NY: Anchor Books, 1987)

Schneidman, Edwin. *Death: Current Perspectives* (CA: Mayfield Publication Co., 1984)

Schwartz, Enid. PESI HealthCare seminar entitled: *Understanding and Effectively Managing End-of-Life Issues* (WI: PSI HealthCare, 2001)

Seale, Alan. *Intuitive Living: A Sacred Path* (Boston: Weiser Books, 1997)

Chapter 8 – Beyond Remembering

Kauffman, Stuart. *At Home in the Universe: The Search for the Laws of Self-Organization and Complexity* (Oxford: Oxford University Press, 1995)

SELECTED RESOURCES

Alzheimer's and Other Dementias

Bahr, M. *The Memory Box* (IL: A. Whitman & Company, 1992)
[A beautifully written book for children ages 7-11 depicting tender relationships with a grandparent with Alzheimer's and offering imaginative suggestions for positive action.]

Bell, Virginia and David Troxel. *The Best Friends Approach to Alzheimer's Care* (Baltimore: Health Professions Press; Rev. ed., 2003)
[This book presents the Best Friends Model of Care, defining many of the ingredients for interacting with the person instead of the disease.]

Brawley, Elizabeth C. *Designing for Alzheimer's Disease: Strategies for Creating a Better Care Environment* (New York: John Wiley and Sons, 1997)
[Presentation of design considerations for creating a safe and therapeutic environment for a person with dementia.]

Bryden, Christine. *Dancing with Dementia: My Story of Living Positively with Dementia* (London: Jessica Kingsley Publishers, 2005)
[The author explores how dementia challenges our ideas of personal identity and the process of self-discovery it can bring about. She offers suggestions for care providers about what to do without demeaning the person.]

Burdock, Lydia. *The Sunshine on My Face: A Read-Aloud Book for Memory-Challenged Adults* (MD: Health Professions Press, 2004)
[This very unique 2-lap book is a perfect way for friends and family to communicate with persons with dementia and to find meaningful ways to fill the time during visits. It is wonderful for teens and adults.]

Castleman, Michael, Dolores Gallagher-Thompson, and Matthew Naythons. *There's Still a Person in There: The Complete Guide to Treating and Coping with Alzheimer's* (New York: A Perigee Book, 1999.
[An excellent, comprehensive, optimistic and comforting resource.]

Coste, Joanne Koenig. *Learning to Speak Alzheimer's: A Groundbreaking Approach For Everyone Dealing with the Disease* (Boston: Houghton Mifflin Company, 2004)
[Offers practical tips for enhancing communication between patient and caregiver; presents habilitation model of care.]

Davidson, Ann. *Alzheimer's: A Love Story* (NJ: Birch Lane Press/Carroll Publishing, 1977)
[A moving memoir by the wife of a person diagnosed with Alzheimer's.]

DeBaggio, Thomas. *Losing My Mind: An Intimate Look at Life with Alzheimer's* (New York: Free Press, 2002)
[Extraordinary, insightful and first-person account of a man diagnosed with Alzheimer's.]

DeBaggio, Thomas. *When it Gets Dark: An Enlightened Reflection on Life with Alzheimer's* (New York: Free Press, 2003)
[The continuation of author's experience and insights.]

Fazio, Sam, Dorothy Seman, and Jane Stansell. *Rethinking Alzheimer's Care* (Baltimore: Health Professions Press, 1999)

[An excellent resource predominantly for care professionals, which encourages reframing the Alzheimer's experience; includes thought-provoking exercises that explore and implement person-centered caring.]

Feil, Naomi. *The Validation Breakthrough: Simple Techniques for Communicating with People with "Alzheimer's-Type Dementia"* (Baltimore: Health Professions Press; 2nd ed., 2002)

[Presents case studies that illustrate effective techniques that are appropriate when communicating with the person with Alzheimer's disease at the earlier stages of the disease process; emphasis on validation of feelings.]

Fox, Mem. *Wilfred Gordon McDonald Partridge* (CA: Kane/Miller Book Publishers, 1989)

[This wonderful, offbeat, beautifully illustrated book is about a little boy who lives next to a retirement home. It shows the capacity of children to help the elderly remember, and it is particularly notable in its non-patronizing focus on the elderly. It is written for children ages 4-8.]

Glenner, Joy A., et. al. *When Your Loved One Has Dementia: A Simple Guide for Caregivers* (MD: Johns Hopkins University Press, 2005)

[The book looks at the family-caregiver-person with dementia relationship and emphasizes communication, understanding, acceptance and personal growth through the caregiving experience.]

Gray-Davidson, Frena. *The Alzheimer's Sourcebook for Caregivers: A Practical Guide For Getting Through the Day* (IL: Lowell House, 1999)

[This book is written to help family members understand healthy caregiving, discover meaning and purpose in their caregiving, and develop more effective ways to deal with difficult situations and identify solutions.]

Guthrie, D. *Grandpa Doesn't Know It's Me* (New York: Human Sciences Press, 1986)

[A book written for children ages 4-8 that helps describe the symptoms and effects of Alzheimer's disease.]

Hamdy, Ronald, et al., eds. *Alzheimer's Disease: A Handbook for Caregivers* (St. Louis: Mosby; 3rd ed., 1998)

[This book bridges information from interdisciplinary experts and family members. It is particularly helpful in offering practical information about the day to day care as well as practical ideas and solutions for finding support and local resources.]

Laminack, Lester. *The Sunsets of Miss Olivia Wiggins* (GA: Peachtree Publishers, 1998)

[This story reassures the reader that older persons can have a full inner life and will understand the importance of others visiting them. It also speaks to the value of maintaining loving relationships. Written for ages 9-12.]

Mace, Nancy L. and Peter V. Rabins. *The 36-Hour Day: A Family Guide for Caring for Persons with Alzheimer's Disease, Related Dementing Illnesses, and*

Memory Loss in Later Life (NY: Warner Books; Rev. ed., 1999)

[Considered the bible of resources since its initial publication in 1981.]

Snyder, Lisa. *Speaking our Minds: Personal Reflections from Individuals with Alzheimer's* (NY: W. H. Freeman, 2000)

[The author has a discussion with seven persons about how they have coped with the disease and provides some of her own experiences as a caregiver.]

Visiting Nurses Association of America. *Caregiver's Handbook: A Complete Guide To Home Health Care by the Visiting Nurses Association of America* (NY: DK Publishing, Inc., 1998)

[This is a handbook written for those who are caring for the sick or the elderly. It offers practical suggestions and includes good illustrations of caregiving techniques and equipment.]

Warner, M. L. *The Complete Guide to Alzheimer's-Proofing Your Home* (Indiana: Purdue University Press; Revised edition, 2000)

[A good resource for ideas in creating a safe and workable home environment.]

Videos

Iris. Judi Dench, Jim Broadbent, and Kate Winslet. (Available in VHS and DVD: BBC, Intermedia Films, Mirage Enterprises, and Miramax Films; 2001)

[This is a powerful true story of novelist Iris Murdoch and her husband John Bayley from their student days through her battle with Alzheimer's disease. It portrays the devastation of the disease process as well as the power of a loving relationship.]

Marvin's Room. Meryl Streep, Diane Keaton, and Leonardo DiCaprio. (Available in VHS and DVD: Miramax Films; 1996)

[This excellent film looks at the loving relationship between an adult daughter and her father who has a dementing illness. The film highlights shifting family dymanics and relationships around problem solving care issues.]

Sensory Stimulation

Hospice of the Valley's Dementia Program has created the SOS™ (Stimulation of Senses) bag which contains items to help caregivers explore different ways to make meaningful connections. The bags are not sold, since they are easy to replicate, but the Hospice will share the list of items, how to use them and contact information for vendors they used to purchase items. In this way, families can customize whatever tastes, sounds, lotions, scents, books, etc. to maximize the experiences and comfort of their loved ones. For information about creating your own SOS™ bag, send an email to: *dementiaprogrm@hov.org* or call directly to 602-636-6363.

Organizations to Know About

Alzheimer's Association
225 N. Michigan Avenue, Fl. 17
Chicago, IL 60601-7633
(312) 335-8700 or
(800) 272-3900 – Toll free 24 hour Contact Center
www.alz.org
  [The leading organization in the field that has a very user friendly web site; information on the disease, local chapters, multiple services and resources supporting families and caregivers of people with Alzheimer's disease.]

Alzheimer's Disease Education and Referral Center (ADEAR)
ADEAR Center
Box 8250
Silver Spring, MD 20907-8250
(301) 495-3334 or
(800) 438-4380
www.alzheimers.org
  [Has a web site that is now integrated as part of the National Institute on Aging; order publications, search for clinical trials and literature, sign up for email alerts, link to information and referrals.]

Family Caregiver Alliance
180 Montgomery Street, Ste 1100
San Francisco, CA 94104
(415) 434-3388 or
(800) 445-8106
www.caregiver.org
  [A national nonprofit organization that provides education, multiple resources and advocacy to help support and sustain caregivers of individuals who are chronically ill and elderly.]

National Family Caregivers Association
10400 Connecticut Avenue, Suite 500
Kensington, MD 20895-3944
(800) 896-3650
www.nfcacares.org
  [Provides education, support, empowerment and advocacy for family caregivers.]

Inspiration/Nourishment

Albom, Mitch. *Tuesdays with Morrie: An Old Man, a Young Man, and Life's Greatest Lessons* (NY: Broadway Books; Reprint edition, 2002)
  [This simple, universally touching story is about a twinkling-eyed mensch who, even on his deathbed, teaches all about living robustly and fully.

Burnett, Frances H. *The Secret Garden* (NY: HarperTrophy; Reprint ed., 1998)
[This is a book for children of all ages. It weaves the "magical" or spiritual side of things with a fairy tale of two neglected children who reach greater health and wisdom by the help of "magic," some good simple people and a tragedy greater than themselves.]

Chödrön, Pema. *When Things Fall Apart: Heart Advice for Difficult Times* (Boston: Shambala Publications, Inc., 1977)
[Written in a graceful, conversational tone, Chödrön writes about how Tibetan Buddhism can help readers cope with the difficult realities of modern life. Many people felt it helpful in reshaping their perspective on life.]

Davis, Maggie Steincrohn. *Caring in Remembered Ways* (ME: Heartsong Books, 1999)
[This book is an inspiring collection of anecdotes and meditations that honors the deep-seeing ways that the heart knows. It is pure nourishment for the heart.]

Gawain, Shakti and Denise Grimshaw. *Reflections in the Light: Daily Thoughts and Affirmations* (CA: Nataraj Publishing; 2nd edition, 2003)
[This book gives readers an inspirational thought, a useful tool or just some inspirational food for thought each day. Each entry has a heading, a short message or meditation and an affirmation.]

Gibran, Kahlil. *The Prophet* (NY: Knopf Publishing Group, 1923)
[This classic collection of poems and essays on love, marriage, joy, sorrow, and much more has inspired thousands of readers. The concise poetic statements of Gibran's truth and wisdom are free of dogma, power structures and metaphysics.]

Halberstam, Yitta and Judith Leventhal. *Small Miracles: Extraordinary Coincidences From Everyday Life* (MA: Adams Media Corporation, 1997)
[This book is a collection of moving, heartwarming and inspirational stories containing profound teachings, important moral lessons and even what some people call divine messages.]

Hayward, Susan. *A Guide for the Advanced Soul: A Book of Insight* (Australia: Hayward Books; 1999)
[This little book is filled with wisdom, knowledge and comforting quotes from Rumi, Emerson, Rilke, Goeth and Whitman. Each page has a different quotation for reflection, guidance and/or inspiration.]

Lamott, Anne. *Traveling Mercies: Some Thoughts in Faith* (IA: Anchor Publications, 2000)
[Several people recommended this as a very delightful, funny and touching collection of essays describing the author's reluctant journey into faith. It is a spiritual writing that wonderfully uses concrete language, solid scenes and believable metaphors—mixing some irreverence in with her wit.]

Moore, Thomas. *Care of the Soul: A Guide for Cultivating Depth and Sacredness in Everyday Life* (NY: HarperCollins Publ., 1992)
[This book is considered by many to be one of the best primers for soul work ever written. Moore encourages the reader to nurture the soul in everyday life

and shows how to cultivate dignity, peace and depth of character.]

Rushnell, Squire D. *When God Winks: How the Power of Coincidence Guides Your Life* (NY: Atria Books, 2002)

[The author provides a collection of confounding coincidences and encourages the reader to consider that recognition of synchronicities can be used to vastly improve our lives.]

Zukav, Gary. *Thoughts from the Seat of the Soul: Meditations for Souls in Process* (NY: Fireside, 2001)

[This spiral bound collection of 280 thoughts (inspired by his bestseller *The Seat of the Soul*) is said to be packaged like a one-a-day vitamin. Some people found the quotations helpful throughout the day for spiritual guidance and reflection.]

Expanding Awareness and Intuition

Childre, Doc and Howard Martin. *The HeartMath Solution* (San Francisco: HarperCollins Publishers, 1999)

[This book provides comprehensive information, helpful tools and techniques to access your heart intelligence.]

Childre, Doc and Deborah Rozman. *Transforming Stress: The HeartMath Solution for Relieving Worry, Fatigue, and Tension* (CA: New Harbinger Publications, Inc., 2005)

[This book leads the reader through a step-by-step process to release stress and anxiety in order to transform that energy into peaceful, creative energy. It presents many helpful tools for learning how to live authentically from the heart.]

Chödrön, Pema and Frans Lanting, photographer. *Pema Chödrön: Awakening the Heart* (Amber Lotus;2006)

[This 2007 calendar features quotes from Ms. Chödrön's book *Comfortable with Uncertainty*, which is designed to help cultivate compassion and awareness in daily challenges. These quotations are paired with the beautiful and meditative nature photography of Frans Lanting.]

Goldstein, Joseph and Jack Kornfield. *Seeking the Heart of Wisdom* (MA: Shambhala Publications, 2001)

[This classic text is a rich source of Buddhist wisdom and practice. It is an introductory guide that contains valuable exercises and offers trusted advice about working through the "difficulties and hindrances" that may arise while practicing.]

Kabat-Zinn, Jon, *Wherever You Go, There You Are: Mindfulness Meditation in Everyday Life* (New York: Hyperion, 1994)

[For those who are drawn to meditation for the first time and to longtime practitioners, this book is a very clear and practical guide for reclaiming the ability to be fully present and to experience the richness of each moment.]

Millman, Dan. *No Ordinary Moments: A Peaceful Warrior's Guide to Daily Life* (CA: H. J. Kramer Inc., 1992)

[Written in a straightforward, everyday manner, this book contains exercises to help balance the body, liberate the mind, accept our emotions and open our hearts.]

Nelson, Martia. *Coming Home: The Return to True Self* (CA: New World Library, 1993)
[Nelson offers simple suggestions for helping us integrate our human experience with our essential spiritual nature so we can express our full potential.]

Pearsall, Paul. *The Hearts Code* (NY: Broadway Books, 1999)
[Documenting the stories he tells with medical and psychological literature, the author shows how the human heart, not the brain, holds the secrets that link body, mind and spirit.]

Prather, Hugh. *The Little Book of Letting Go: A Revolutionary 30-day Program to Cleanse your Mind, Lift your Spirit and Replenish your Soul* (ME: Conari Press, 2000)
[The author brings wit, wisdom, insight and practical help into facilitating the process of "letting go" of some difficult attachments while offering ways to lift the soul to its maximum capabilities.]

Rosanoff, Nancy. *Intuition Workout: A Practical Guide to Discovering and Developing Your Inner Knowing* (CT: Aslan Publishing, 1991)
[A step-by-step, thought-by-thought 'how to' guide for reaching and developing one's latent intuitive capabilities.]

Seale, Alan. *Intuitive Living: A Sacred Path* (ME: Weiser Books, 2001)
[A gentle workbook that assumes an open curiosity about the basic tools of the spiritual life: meditation, journaling, body work, prayer, mindfulness and visualization.]

Shapiro, E. & D. *Clear Mind Open Heart: Healing Yourself, Your Relationships, and the Planet* (CA: The Crossing Press, 1998)
[This book teaches us how we can overcome our fear and guilt, experience loving relationships with ourselves and others, and use relaxation for magic and joy.]

Tolle, Eckart. *The Power of Now: A Guide to Spiritual Enlightenment* (CA: New World Library, 1999)
[The author's message is simple: living in the now is the truest path to happiness and enlightenment. While this message may not seem stunningly original or fresh, the writing is clear, and the voice is supportive and enthusiastic.]

Virtue, Doreen. *Divine Guidance: How to Have a Dialogue with God and Your Guardian Angels* (LA: Renaissance Books, 1998)
[This book offers practical instruction in how to open your mind and free your heart and soul to receive communications from God and the angels; it maps out several clairvoyant styles and helps readers identify which style is their own.]

Walsh, Roger. *Essential Spirituality: The 7 Central Practices to Awaken Heart and Mind* (NY: John Wiley & Sons, Inc., 1999)
[This book identifies and brings together the shared practices found in the world's religions and presents them in a very down-to-earth way, providing exercises that are simple, straightforward and effective.]

Zukav, Gary and Linda Francis. *The Heart of the Soul: Emotional Awareness* (NY: Free Press, 2002)
[Drawing on Hindu and Buddhist thought, Taoism, Christianity, psychology and many other sources, the authors encourage readers to journey from their head to their heart in order to "empower the soul" through numerous exercises and activities.]

Healing/Healing Touch

Berkson, Devaki. *The Foot Book: Healing the Body Through Foot Reflexology* (San Francisco: HarperCollins Publishers, 1992)
[This book is a holistic guide to healing, integrating the use of reflexology, yoga, nutrition, herbology, acupuncture/acupressure and imagery/meditation and exercise.]

Brennan, Barbara. *Hands of Light: A Guide to Healing Through the Human Energy Field* (NY: Bantam Books, 1988)
[A scientist looks at bioenergetic healing and offers specific techniques for expanding the perceptual tools of healing, seeing auras and spiritual healing.]

Dreamhealer, Adam. *Dreamhealer 2 Guide to Self-Empowerment* (Dreamhealer.com, 2004)
[Several people said that the information provided about energetic healing is inspiring while broken down into its simplest and purest form. There is some redundancy, but with simple and easy to understand instructions on how to clear your mind and see auras.]

Feltman, John (editor). *Hands on Healing: Massage Remedies for Hundreds of Health Problems* (PA: Rodale Press, 1991)
[This book takes a look at popular to obscure forms of therapies which focus on the healing power of physical contact. It provides a lively account of the background and theory, potential benefits, and interviews.]

Harper, Tom. *The Uncommon Touch: An Investigation of Spiritual Healing* (Ontario: McClelland & Stewart, Inc., 1994)
[An examination of the phenomenon of spiritual healing from a more scientific perspective.]

Krieger, Dolores. *Accepting Your Power to Heal: The Personal Practice of Therapeutic Touch* (VT: Bear & Company, 1993)
[Clear and easy to follow, this book encourages us to acknowledge our innate healing abilities and provides experiential exercises to teach basic Therapeutic Touch techniques.]

Miles, Pamela. *Reiki: A Comprehensive Guide* (NY: J. P.Tarcher, 2006)
[Written in a language that is accessible to both the general public and seasoned professionals; this is an invaluable resource whether you have been attuned to Reiki or are simply exploring the possibility of learning more about this system of healing and spiritual development.]

Thei, John F. and Matthew Thei. *Touch for Health* (CA: DeVorss & Company, 20050
[This updated edition of Thei's 1973 practical guide to natural health

uses acupressure touch and massage. It is concise, easy to understand, nicely illustrated and easy to put in practice.]

Sanford, Agnes. *The Healing Gifts of the Spirit* (San Francisco: Harper & Row, 1984)

[A step-by-step approach to spiritual healing that reflects the author's personal experience of the restorative power of prayer. It is a reliable and inspiring handbook for developing our innate capacity for richer living and giving through the healing gifts of the Spirit.]

Healing Sounds

Evenson, Dean & Soundings Ensemble. *Sound Healing* (Soundings of the Planets, 1998) This CD can be ordered at *www.PeaceThroughMusic.com* or through Amazon.

[What sets this CD apart from others of its ilk is that the pieces are musically strong and enjoyable to listen to. It is excellent accompaniment to simple relaxation, any healing treatment or meditation.]

Fu, Grandmaster Wei Zhong. *Emei Sacred Healing Sounds: For Healthy Internal Organs* (International Qigong Association, 2003) This CD can be ordered from visiting the Emei Qigong website: *www.emeiqigong.com*.

[This CD contains several healing sounds made by this Qigong master which are said to be universal codes, the vibrations of which unlock healing energy and bring it down to this dimension.]

Hospice of the Valley's Dementia Program sells sing-along CD's in English, Spanish and Hebrew/Yiddish for only $5.00 (to simply cover the cost of shipping and handling). To order, send an email to: *dementiaprogrm@hov.org* or call directly at 602-636-6363.

[They will also forward lyrics and a guide to using music most effectively for persons with advanced dementia. A current project is to slowly receite the 23rd Psalm over calming music for persons with advanced dementia.]

Various Artists. *Classical Spirit* (LIND Institute, 1999) This CD can only be ordered directly from Archedigm, Inc. Order on-line by sending an e-mail to *info@archedigm.com* or send your request to Archedigm, Inc., P.O. Box 1109, Olney, MD 20830-1109.

[This program of chants and choral masterpieces from the 12th century to the 20th century was designed by Linda Keiser Mardis. Many family members have found this CD helpful for their own relaxation and revitalization.]

Various Artists. *Harp Adagios: Over Two Hours of the World's Most Relaxing Music.* (Decca, 2005). *Amazon.com*.

[Available at Amazon.com, this CD is just one of many in the Decca Adagio series—all providing an excellent choice of pieces and a very good quality of performers. These slower paced pieces are soothing for persons with dementia and care providers alike.]

Various Artists. *Relax with the Classics* Series (LIND Institute, 1996) Various CDs from this series can be ordered at *www.relaxwiththeclassics.com* or by calling 1.800.LEARN.R.US.

[Recent studies show that the beautifully soothing music in the *Largo* and *Adagio* CDs provide numerous health and wellness benefits, reduce verbally and physically agitated behaviors in persons with Alzheimer's and are highly recommended for reducing stress. Their CDs entitled *Pastorale, Andante,* and are also highly beneficial.]

INDEX

V

W

CARD CUT & CARRY

Laminate this business card-size reminder of the 6 **IF LOST** concepts/principles for creating connections, and it will always be accessible for easy reference.

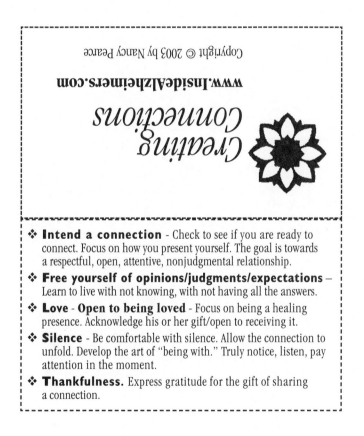

Copyright © 2003 by Nancy Pearce

www.InsideAlzheimers.com

Creating Connections

- ❖ **Intend a connection** - Check to see if you are ready to connect. Focus on how you present yourself. The goal is towards a respectful, open, attentive, nonjudgmental relationship.
- ❖ **Free yourself of opinions/judgments/expectations** – Learn to live with not knowing, with not having all the answers.
- ❖ **Love** - **Open to being loved** - Focus on being a healing presence. Acknowledge his or her gift/open to receiving it.
- ❖ **Silence** - Be comfortable with silence. Allow the connection to unfold. Develop the art of "being with." Truly notice, listen, pay attention in the moment.
- ❖ **Thankfulness.** Express gratitude for the gift of sharing a connection.